VIROLOGY MONOGRAPHS

DIE VIRUSFORSCHUNG IN EINZELDARSTELLUNGEN

CONTINUING/FORTFÜHRUNG VON
HANDBOOK OF VIRUS RESEARCH
HANDBUCH DER VIRUSFORSCHUNG
FOUNDED BY/BEGRÜNDET VON
R. DOERR

EDITED BY/HERAUSGEGEBEN VON

S. GARD · C. HALLAUER · K. F. MEYER

5

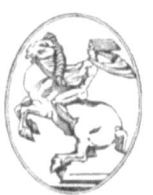

1969

SPRINGER-VERLAG

WIEN · NEW YORK

HERPES SIMPLEX AND PSEUDORABIES VIRUSES

BY

A. S. KAPLAN

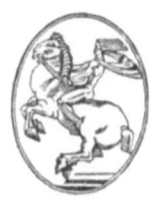

1969

SPRINGER-VERLAG

WIEN · NEW YORK

ISBN-13: 978-3-7091-8231-4   e-ISBN-13: 978-3-7091-8229-1
DOI: 10.1007/978-3-7091-8229-1

Herpes Simplex and Pseudorabies Viruses

By

A. S. Kaplan

Department of Microbiology, Research Laboratories
Albert Einstein Medical Center
Philadelphia, Pennsylvania, U.S.A.

With 14 Figures

Table of Contents

I. Introduction

The herpes group consists of viruses which have been placed together on the basis of a number of distinguishing features that they share in common (ANDREWES, 1962). All these viruses are relatively large, possess identical morphological characteristics, contain DNA, and are extremely sensitive to inactivation by ether; these viruses are also assembled within the nucleus of the host cell and induce the formation of eosinophilic intranuclear inclusions. The epidemiology of some of the best known viruses in this group (herpes simplex, pseudorabies, and B-virus) is also similar (BURNET et al., 1939). Herpes simplex virus exists in the latent state in man, the natural host for this virus, and becomes overt in individuals subject to some form of stress; this condition appears to be paralleled by pseudorabies virus in its natural host, swine and by B-virus in monkeys. In each instance, transmission of the virus to a susceptible host other than the natural one results usually in marked symptoms and death.

This chapter is confined to a description of herpes simplex and pseudorabies viruses; B-virus is described separately elsewhere in the Handbook. Since the clinical aspects of the diseases caused by herpes simplex virus and pseudorabies virus have been well described, greater emphasis will be placed, therefore, on the basic biological and biochemical properties of these viruses; their clinical features will be discussed only briefly. Furthermore, since host-virus interactions at the cellular level can be analyzed quantitatively, studies on the interactions of the viruses and their host cells that have been made with cells cultivated *in vitro* will be examined in preference to studies performed with animals.

II. History

A. Herpes Simplex Virus

BESWICK (1962) has traced the origin of the name, herpes, which has been used in medicine for at least 25 centuries. Hippocrates, for example, used herpes to describe certain kinds of diseases of the skin and although herpes labialis (febrilis) may have been included in the diseases known as herpes by Hippocrates, it certainly was not the only or principal condition to which he gave this name. A clear account of herpes febrilis was first given in England in the 17th century, and the first adequate description of this virus under its modern name was made in the 18th century. However, not until the end of the 19th century was the modern concept of the virus and the disease it causes finally accepted.

VIDAL (1873) was probably the first to show that herpes febrilis was infectious. However, there was little interest in this finding, until after World War I when LÖWENSTEIN (1919) published evidence that herpes keratitis and labialis yielded a virus that would produce characteristic lesions on the cornea of a rabbit. LÖWENSTEIN had confirmed essentially earlier experiments by GRÜTER who had not published his findings. Later, GRÜTER (1920) published experiments in which he showed that the virus could be passaged successfully from an experimentally infected rabbit to the cornea of a blind man.

The appearance of intranuclear inclusion bodies in infected cells characteristic of infections with herpes simplex virus was first described by LIPSCHÜTZ (1921). Although there was some dispute at that time about the nature of these structures,

there seemed little doubt that they contained virus after experiments by BAUM-
GARTNER (1935) who isolated the inclusions by micromanipulation and found
that herpes keratitis could be reproduced by a single, washed inclusion.

A great deal of interest in herpes simplex virus was generated by the discovery
that it would produce encephalitis in rabbits (DOERR, 1920), as well as by the
isolation of a virus with the characteristics of herpes simplex by LEVADITI and
HARVIER (1920) from a patient who had succumbed to von Economo's encephalitis, a disease that had reached epidemic proportions. These reports fostered
the notion that herpes simplex virus might be the causative agent of this disease;
however, this notion proved to be incorrect, even though herpes simplex is one
of the viruses that can cause human encephalitis.

About twenty years later, the position of herpes simplex virus as an infectious
agent was questioned by DOERR (1938), because the virus did not appear to
move from one individual to another and seemed to be generated endogenously
by individuals after nonspecific stimuli. The discovery by ANDREWES and CAR-
MICHAEL (1930) that most normal adults in the population possess neutralizing
antibodies against herpes simplex virus in their blood, and that recurrent herpes
infection develops only in those patients with neutralizing antibodies also seemed
inconsistent with the concept that the virus was a cause of disease, since this
is contrary to the usual virus-host interaction in which an immune individual
does not develop disease. The role of herpes simplex virus as a disease-producing
agent was elucidated by DODD et al. (1938) who showed that herpes simplex
virus could be isolated repeatedly from the mouths of infants with a common
form of acute vesicular stomatitis and by BURNET and WILLIAMS (1939) who
demonstrated that (1) infants developed neutralizing antibodies during the
periods of convalescence from vesicular stomatitis, and that (2) herpes simplex
infections appear to persist for life and that virus can be isolated from individuals
with recurrent infections. Succeeding investigations showed also that herpes
simplex could be isolated from a number of infections such as eczema
herpeticum, vulvovaginitis, keratoconjunctivitis, and meningoencephalitis, and
it was soon recognized that primary infection by herpes simplex virus is common
in man and that after recovery the virus appears to enter into a latent state.

B. Pseudorabies Virus

The disease caused by pseudorabies virus has been recognized for a long
time, and descriptions of illness in cattle characteristic of infections with this
virus appeared in the United States in the first quarter of the 19th century
(HANSON, 1954). This disease, called "Mad Itch" in the United States because
of the vigorous rubbing of their affected parts by diseased cattle, was also prevalent in other parts of the world and first shown by AUJESZKY (1902) in Hungary
to be due to a virus. Because of certain clinical aspects, there was at first some
confusion about the relation of this virus to rabies, whence the name pseudorabies, but it was soon found that the two viruses are not related. AUJESZKY studied
pseudorabies thoroughly and recognized by most criteria that it is a virus, however, he did not succeed in proving that it could be passed through a bacterial
filter. This was accomplished later by SCHMIEDHOFER (1910) and SANGIORGI
(1914).

Shortly after pseudorabies virus was discovered, MAREK (1904) termed the disease "Infectious Bulbar Paralysis" because in rabbits the medullary centers are very susceptible to the virus and under certain conditions, only the medulla appears to be affected. However, in other animals (monkeys and swine) there is no particular susceptibility of the medulla to pseudorabies virus and the name "Infectious Bulbar Paralysis" is not a particularly apt description of the disease.

In 1931, SHOPE showed that the "mad itch" appearing in cattle in Iowa was the same as the disease described by AUJESZKY and that the two viruses are immunologically identical (SHOPE, 1932).

III. Classification and Nomenclature

There have been a number of attempts to classify related viruses into groups that have evolutionary and phylogenetic relationships. These attempts have proved difficult and none has been accepted universally.

Some of the earlier formal attempts to develop a satisfactory basis for virus taxonomy have been summarized by ANDREWES (1962) who also formulated a "fundamental" set of criteria for virus classification as follows: (1) type of viral nucleic acid (DNA or RNA); (2) size; (3) number of capsomeres; (4) presence or absence of a viral membrane; (5) cellular site of virus multiplication (cytoplasmic or nuclear); (6) site of maturation; (7) sensitivity to ether. In addition to these so-called fundamental criteria, other, less stable, criteria were also used to aid in the classification of the viruses: (1) natural methods of transmission; (2) host, tissue, and cell tropism; (3) pathology. According to these criteria, the herpesviruses constitute a main group that is composed of relatively large, ether-sensitive, DNA viruses, which develop within the cell nucleus and acquire a membrane on passage into the cytoplasm. This group of viruses also induces the formation of eosinophilic intranuclear inclusions. In this classification, the viruses were given binomial names. Thus, herpes simplex virus, which is indigenous to man, was named *Herpesvirus hominis*, and pseudorabies virus, which is indigenous to swine, *Herpesvirus suis*.

TOURNIER and LWOFF (1966) have proposed a classification which retains some of the features of ANDREWES' taxonomic arrangement but is far more formal in design. In the TOURNIER-LWOFF scheme, viruses are classified on the basis of the following criteria: (1) type of nucleic acid (DNA or RNA); (2) symmetry of the nucleocapsid; (3) presence or absence of an envelope; and (4), for cubical viruses, the number of triangulations and the number of capsomeres (or morphological units). Pseudorabies and herpes simplex are viruses that contain DNA within cubical nucleocapsids surrounded by an outer membrane or envelope; the nucleocapsids are icosahedral with a triangulation number of 16 and consist of 162 capsomeres. Thus, according to this system of classification, pseudorabies and herpes simplex viruses belong to the subphylum, *Deoxyvira;* class, *Deoxycubica;* family, *Herpesviridae;* genus, *Herpesvirus;* and species, *suis* and *hominis*, respectively.

Another proposal for the classification of viruses has been made which is based on a nonhierarchal approach and consists of cryptograms composed of four symbols (WILDY, 1966). For herpes simplex virus, this cryptogram would be as follows: $\frac{D}{2} : \frac{68}{*} : \frac{S}{S} : \frac{V}{O}$, the symbols indicating that this virus contains double-stranded DNA with a molecular weight of 68 million, the per cent composition of the DNA is unknown (indicated by the asterisk), the viral particle and its nucleocapsid are spherical, and finally the virus has a vertebrate host but no known vector. The cryptogram for pseudorabies virus is identical, except that the molecular weight of its DNA is slightly higher.

It has been suggested also (MELNICK and McCOMBS, 1966) that the herpes viruses should be further divided into two subgroups on the basis of whether the viruses are readily released from cells in an infectious form (group A) or whether they are mostly cell-associated and can be detected only with difficulty, if at all (group B). According to this suggestion, herpes simplex and pseudorabies viruses would belong to group A; the varicella-herpes zoster viruses and cytomegaloviruses would belong to group B.

IV. Properties of the Viruses
A. Morphology
1. Size

The size of viral particles may be determined by indirect, physical methods or by direct observation in an electron microscope. Herpes simplex and pseudorabies viruses have been examined by the various techniques and have been found to range in diameter from 110 mμ to 230 mμ (Table 1). This wide variation in size probably stems from deficiencies inherent in some of the techniques that have been employed.

An early, indirect technique for measuring the size of viruses was devised by ELFORD (ELFORD et al., 1933; ELFORD and GALLOWAY, 1936) who used collodion membrane filters with pre-determined average pore sizes. Although this method is not as sophisticated, nor as accurate as the techniques in current usage, the size determined for herpes simplex virus was not wide of the mark. ELFORD et al. (1933) arrived at a diameter for this virus of about 100 mμ to 150 mμ, which certainly ranges close to that obtained by later, improved techniques (see Table 1). The collodion membrane filter technique was later supplemented by two additional indirect physical methods, namely, diffusion and sedimentation in the ultracentrifuge, particularly the latter technique.

Ultracentrifugal analysis determines the size and mass of the viral particles by their movement in the centrifugal field. This method of analysis is based on a number of assumptions, including a spherical shape for the viral particle, and there is a large element of uncertainty about the estimates this procedure yields on the size of the viruses. Despite these limitations, the estimates of the sizes of herpes simplex virus obtained by this indirect method have been reasonably accurate (see Table 1).

The indirect techniques for the determination of the size of viral particles have been largely supplanted by direct observation by means of electron microscopy which is now the most extensively used technique for the measurement of virus size. In addition to size, observations made with the electron microscope yield information also on the external and internal structure of viruses. The early problem of poor image contrast was overcome by shadow-casting, a technique in which the particles are coated with heavy metals. The size and structural details of the viral particles are even more clearly defined when they are embedded in polymers and are cut into thin-sections before being examined in the electron microscope. The type of polymer used for embedding may alter the shape of the viral particles (see below) and this may account, in part, for the differences in size given in Table 1.

Table 1. *Size of Herpes Simplex and Pseudorabies Viruses*

Virus	Strain	Method of measurement		References
		Electron microscopy mµ	Ultracentrifugation mµ	
Herpes simplex			180—220	BECHHOLD and SCHLESINGER (1933)
		175[1]		CORIELL et al. (1950)
		165[2]		EPSTEIN (1962)
		200—220[1]		EVANS and MELNICK (1949)
	Lennette	150—170[2]		FALKE et al. (1959)
	H 4	184[2]		KAPLAN and VATTER (1959)
		165[2]		LUSE et al. (1965)
		200[2]		MORGAN et al. (1953)
	HRE	110—130[2]		MORGAN et al. (1954)
	JM	120—130[2]		MORGAN et al. (1959)
	Armstrong	116[1]	96	MUNK and ACKERMANN (1953)
	HFEM	135[2]		STOKER et al. (1958)
	HFEM	180[3]		WILDY et al. (1960)
Pseudorabies		170[2]		FELLUGA (1963)
		186[2]		KAPLAN and VATTER (1959)
		150—180[3]		REISSIG and KAPLAN (1962)
	117	170—230[3]		TONEVA (1965)

[1] Shadow-cast.   [2] Thin-section.   [3] Phosphotungstic acid negative stain.

Lately, a new technique, negative staining with phosphotungstic acid, has been used widely and has provided a wealth of information on virus structure (BRENNER and HORNE, 1959). This technique consists of mixing virus preparations with approximately 1% phosphotungstic acid which is neutralized with KOH to pH 7.0 to 7.2. This mixture is sprayed on electron microscope specimen grids and is observed in the electron microscope. The phosphotungstate does not stain the protein or nucleic acid of viral particles, which remain relatively transparent to the electron beam. This method has provided probably the most reliable estimate of the size of herpes simplex and pseudorabies viruses which appear to have a diameter of approximately 180 mµ.

2. Structure

In thin-sections, as well as in negatively-stained preparations, herpes simplex virus (EPSTEIN, 1962a; FALKE et al., 1959; KAPLAN and VATTER, 1959; LUSE et al., 1965; MORGAN et al., 1953, 1954, 1959; STOKER et al., 1958; WILDY et al.,

1960) and pseudorabies virus (KAPLAN and VATTER, 1959; REISSIG and KAPLAN, 1962; FELLUGA, 1963; TONEVA, 1965) are indistinguishable (Figs. 1, 2, and 3).

The general appearance of the viruses in thin-section is dependent to some extent upon the kind of polymers used for embedding the virions and upon

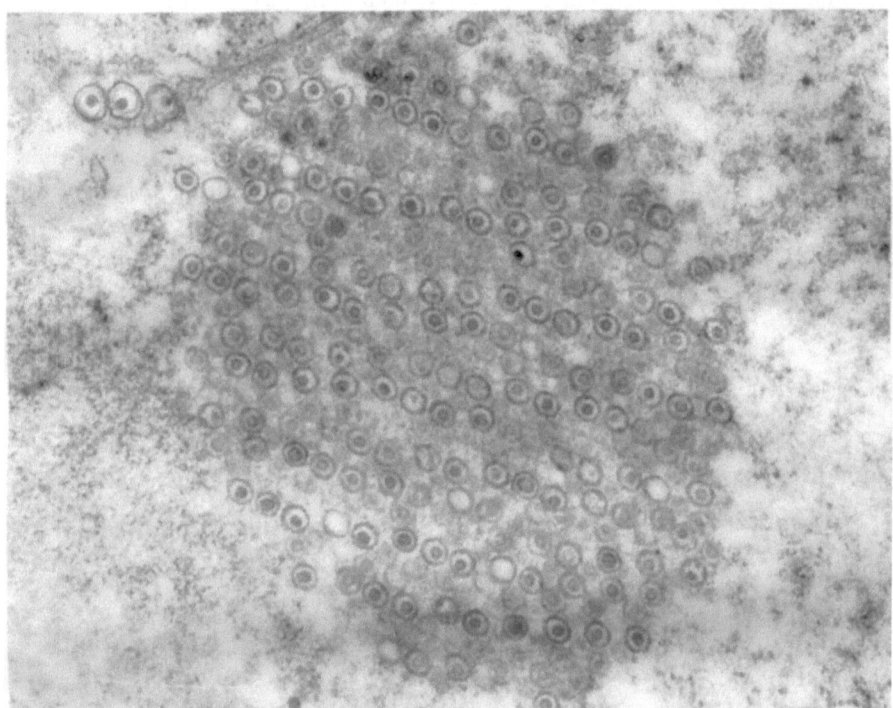

Fig. 1 A. Electron micrograph of a thin-section through a crystal of herpes simplex virus. Note that at the upper left there are three viral particles with double membranes, × 45,000.

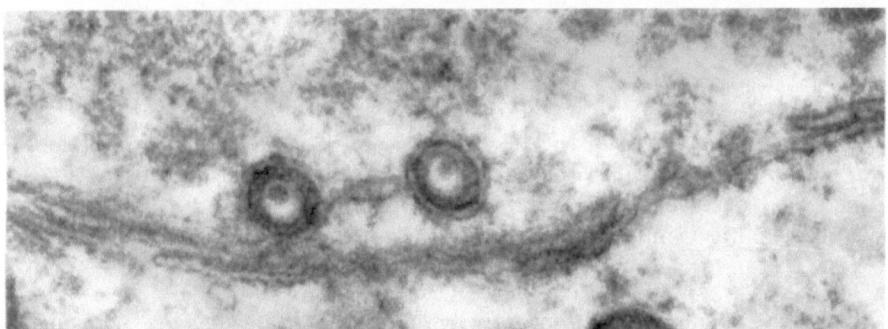

Fig. 1 B. Viral particles with triple membranes. The outermost membrane encloses the virus and appears on the left to be continuous with the nuclear membrane. The cytoplasm is at the bottom. × 87,000. From C. MORGAN et al., J. exp. Med. 110, 643 (1959).

the method of preparing the samples. It was found, for example, that after being embedded in methacrylate, herpes simplex virus was sometimes round but more frequently oval; however, after being embedded in aquon, the viral particles were more frequently spherical or almost so (EPSTEIN, 1962a).

In thin-sections of the viral particles, the electron dense central body, which
is in an eccentric position, may vary in shape and appears round, oval or sometimes like a short ended rod, depending probably on the angle at the time of
sectioning. This central body lies within a zone of lower density, which, in turn,
is surrounded by a double, sometimes triple, membrane, as illustrated in Figs. 1
and 2.

Preparations of herpes simplex and pseudorabies viruses stained negatively
with phosphotungstic acid show the three main components in greater detail (WILDY
et al., 1960; REISSIG and KAPLAN, 1962): (1) A core in the center of the particle
which is most likely equivalent to the electron dense nucleoid observed in thin-
sections of the virus; (2) a capsid surrounding the core (the outer surface of the

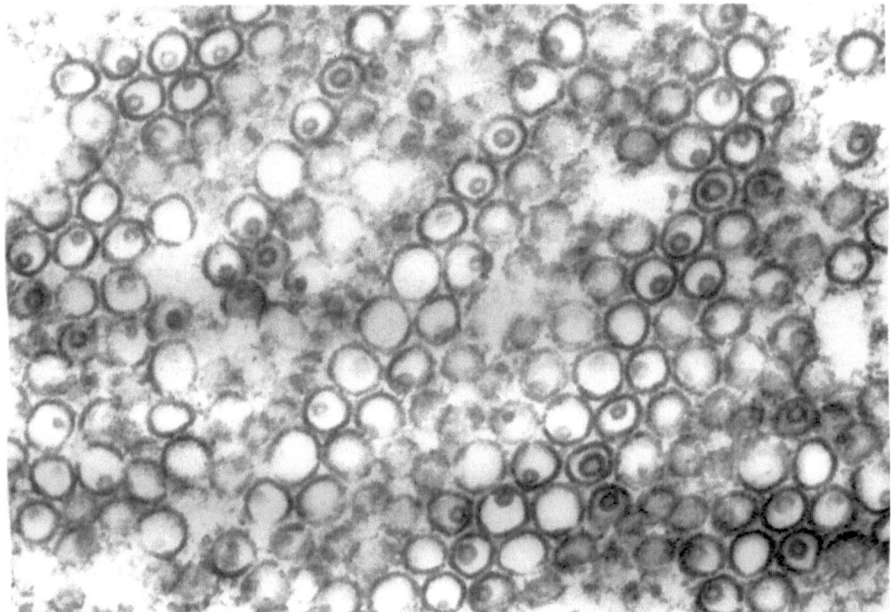

Fig. 2 A.   Electron micrograph of a thin-section through a crystal of pseudorabies virus,   × 73,500.

capsid probably corresponds to the "inner membrane" seen in thin-section);
(3) an outer membrane called the envelope that encloses the capsid (see Fig. 3).
The envelope observed after staining with phosphotungstic acid corresponds
in size to the outer membrane observed in thin-sections of the viruses.

a) Core

This area, as observed in negatively stained preparations, is polygonal,
usually hexagonal, in shape and has, in the case of herpes simplex virus, an
average diameter of about 75 mμ. This size is somewhat larger than the electron
dense central body observed in thin-sections of virions of both herpes simplex
virus (MORGAN et al., 1959; EPSTEIN, 1962a) and of pseudorabies virus (FELLUGA,
1963). The exact composition of the core is not known but there is evidence indicating that the viral nucleic acid is located in this area. This is shown by the
fact that after fixation and thin-sectioning, treatment with DNase removes

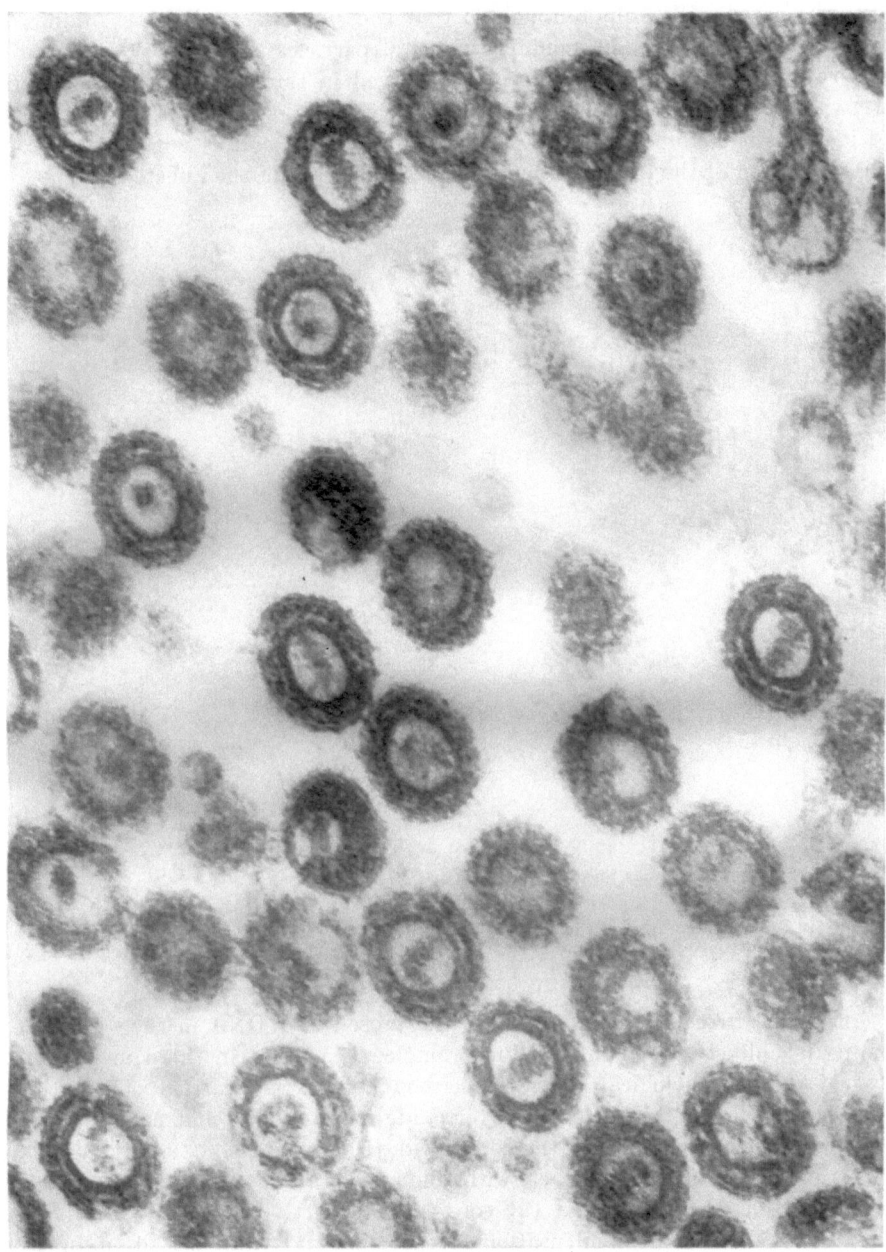

Fig. 2 B.   Extracellular mature viral particles in the extracellular space near the cell wall. Polygonal profiles of the first dense coat are visible in some particles, as well as the indented profile of the third dense coat, × 129,000. From B. FELLUGA, Ann. Sclavo 5, 412 (1963).

the electron dense core, leaving an empty space in the central area of herpes simplex virus (EPSTEIN, 1962a). Furthermore, when pseudorabies virus-infected cells are treated with 5-fluorouracil, so that the synthesis of DNA is inhibited and no viral DNA is made, noninfective viral particles are produced which do not possess the electron dense core, as observed in thin-sections (REISSIG and KAPLAN, 1962). These particles have the same external structure as intact virus and it seems therefore that the DNA contained in the core is not essential for the aggregation of the protein subunits into virus shells in the infected cells.

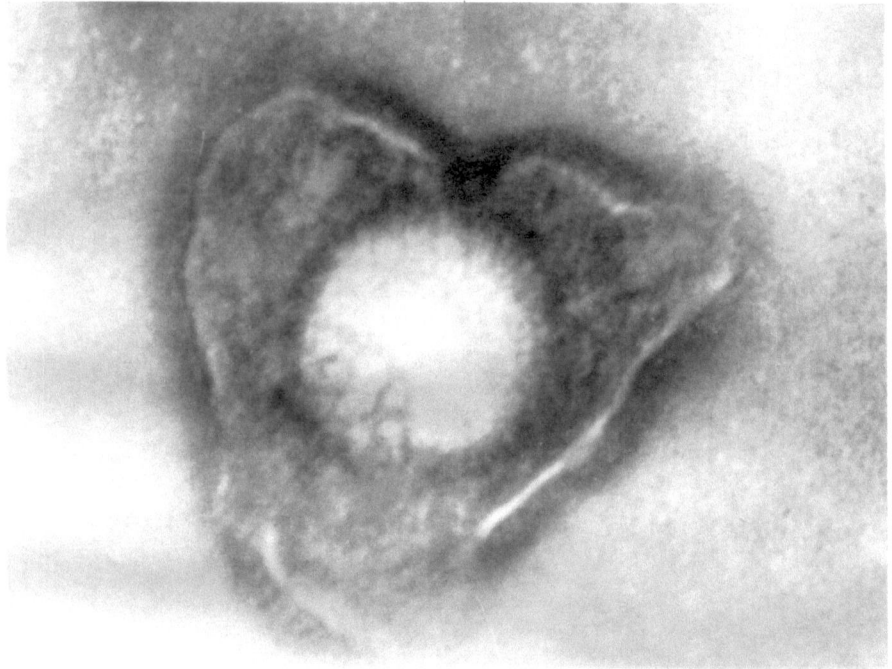

Fig. 3A. Electron micrographs of the viruses stained negatively with phosphotungstic acid. Herpes simplex virus. Note envelope surrounding capsid, ×450,000. From P. WILDY et al., Virology 12, 204 (1960).

Although all the evidence points to the presence of DNA in the viral core, it appears unlikely to be the only macromolecule present in this substructure. Most of the morphological studies described above were carried out in thin-sections of virus fixed with osmium tetroxide, a procedure that contributes to the electron dense character of the core. BAHR (1954) and KELLENBERGER (1960) found that osmium tetroxide reacts with amino acids and therefore stains proteins primarily. It is thus clear that the core consists partly of proteins. The DNA may act as a center of condensation for proteins and thus may be indirectly responsible for the density of the viral core to the electron beam.

That the core may be composed of more than DNA alone is also suggested by a discrepancy between the size of the "radiation-sensitive volume" of the virus (POLLARD, 1954) and the size of the core as measured with the electron microscope. When herpes simplex virus was irradiated with X-rays and the logarithm of surviving virus was plotted as a function of dose, it was found that the sensitive volume of free virus is 22×10^7 Å³ which would correspond to a sphere of 38 mμ in diameter (POWELL, 1959). Using α-rays, BONET-MAURY (1948) calculated a diameter of 32 mμ for the radiation-sensitive volume of herpes simplex virus. According to these results, the radiation-sensitive volume should

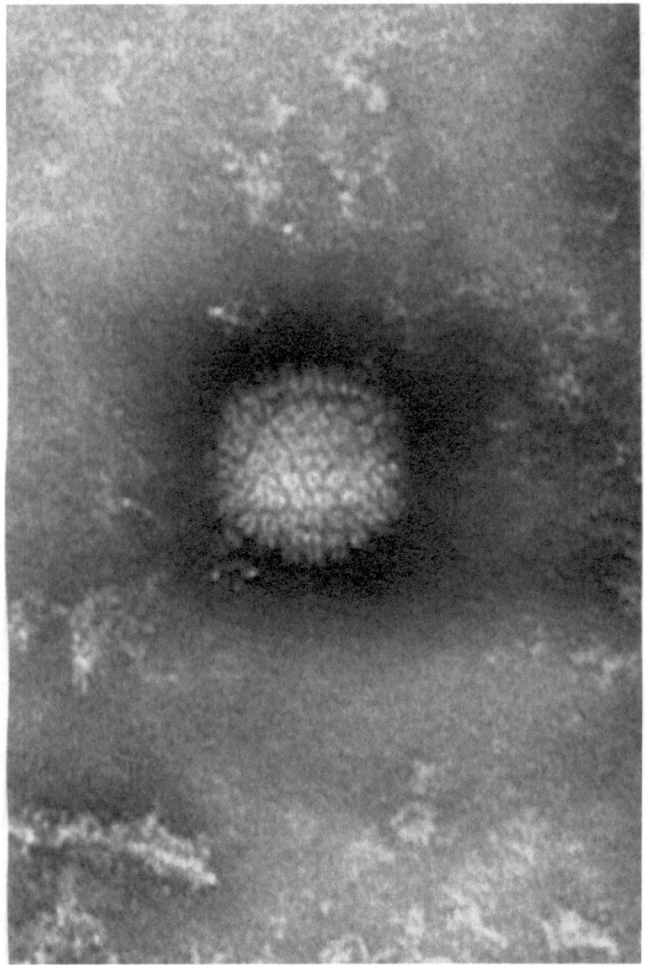

Fig. 3 B. Pseudorabies virus capsid, ×315,000. From M. REISSIG and A. S. KAPLAN, Virology 16, 1 (1962).

occupy about 1% of the total volume of the virus. Because the core occupies a much larger volume (about 6%), WILDY et al. (1960) have concluded that the core contains some other material in addition to DNA. However, the assumption that one can equate the radiation-sensitive volume of the virus with its nucleic acid has been questioned by LURIA (1955), whose analysis has left some doubt as to the validity of the target theory as a means of providing basic information on the structure of viruses.

b) Capsid

The capsids (average diameter, 110 mμ), as observed in the electron microscope after negative staining with phosphotungstic acid, show varying degrees of angularity; they are composed of hollow, elongated, regularly arranged subunits, the capsomeres, which are polygonal in cross section. The capsomeres of herpes simplex virus are approximately 12 to 13.5 mμ long and 9 to 10 mμ wide with a central hole of approximately 4 mμ. Based on the assumption that the capsomeres are composed of protein, the molecular weight of the capsomeres has been calculated to be about 500,000 and the subunits from which they are built would have a molecular weight of about 80,000 to 100,000 (WILDY and HORNE, 1960). It should be emphasized that these subunits need not be equivalent to the crystallographic subunits described by KLUG and CASPAR (1960).

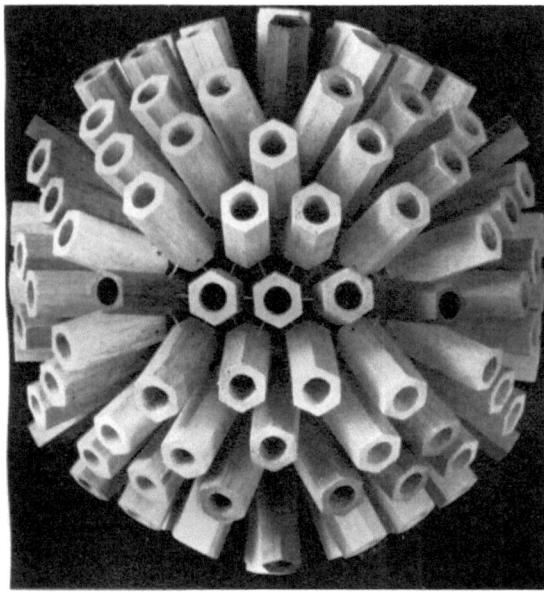

A careful examination of the orderly aligned capsomeres in the capsid revealed that the capsids possess 5:3:2 axial symmetry and have an icosahedral shape. Each edge of the capsid consists of 5 capsomeres. (A body with cubic symmetry has a number of axes of symmetry about which it may be rotated to give a number of identical appearances. An icosahedron, such as herpes simplex virus, which possesses 5:3:2 axial symmetry will, when viewed down a fivefold axis, have five positions in which it can be rotated, each position giving an identical appearance. Similarly, it will have three identical appearances when viewed down a threefold axis, and two identical appearances when viewed down a twofold axis.) The capsid is built from 162 capsomeres (one on each of the twelve fivefold axes, a triad on each of the twenty faces and a triad on each of the thirty edges). It is thought that the overall shape of the capsid is curvilinear and that the faces are domed.

Fig. 4. A model of herpes simplex virus built from 150 hollow hexagonal wooden prisms and 12 hollow pentagonal prisms. This is an icosahedral form. From P. WILDY et al., Virology 12, 204 (1960).

Models have been made of herpes simplex virus based on geometric information presently available. Fig. 4 illustrates such a model which is in the form of an icosahedron; the model is made from 150 hexagonal and 12 pentagonal equally spaced prisms. It is evident from this model that the prisms located on the fivefold and twofold axes are aligned in a radial fashion and that all the prisms in the edges will lie on twofold planes of the icosahedron, while those capsomeres on the faces will be parallel to the axes of threefold symmetry. A spherical model can also be built from the same number of hexagonal and pentagonal prisms arranged in the same manner except that the prisms are at constant radii; the 5:3:2 axial symmetry elements are retained in the spherical form. However, all the data collected thus far indicate that the icosahedral, not the spherical, model is correct.

Incidentally, all the capsomeres, which presumably are composed of protein, appear to be hollow prisms that have five or six sides.

On the examination of the geometry of herpes simplex virus, HORNE and WILDY (1961) derived an empirical formula to describe structures with 5:3:2 symmetry built entirely from hexagons and pentagons. A general formula for the number of capsomeres in capsids with this axial symmetry is $10(n-1)^2+2$, n being the number of capsomeres in each edge shared between the facets of the icosahedron. Thus, because for herpes simplex virus (and for other viruses of this group so far examined, including pseudorabies) $n=5$, there are 162 capsomeres per capsid.

This attempt by HORNE and WILDY (1961) to define mathematically the packing of pentagonal and hexagonal capsomeres to give structures with 5:3:2 symmetry met with limited success, and their empirical approach to the problem has been supplanted by the fuller, more accurate analysis of CASPAR and KLUG (1962) which is based on a consideration of the essential geometric principles involved in icosahedral shell design. A polyhedron whose faces consist of equilateral triangles is called a deltahedron and if it has twenty equilateral triangular faces, it is called an icosahedron. Any icosahedron has 20 T facets, where the triangulation number is given by the rule: $T=Pf^2$, P being any number of the series 1, 3, 7, 13, 19, 21, 31, 37, etc. ($P=h^2+hk+k^2$, for all pairs of integers h and k having no common factor) and f, any integer, 1, 2, 3, 4, etc. For a fixed value of P, increases in f from 1 upward correspond to successive subtriangulations of the deltahedron. The herpesviruses belong to the class, $P=1$. The number of morphological units, M, that would be produced by a clustering of the subunits into hexamers and pentamers is given by the equation $M=10T+2$ or $10(T-1)$ hexamers + 12, and only 12, pentamers. Since the T or triangulation number for the herpes group is 16, there will be 162 morphological units or capsomeres.

c) Envelope

Many of the capsids are enclosed by envelopes of varying shape and size, the diameters fluctuating between 145 and 210 mμ, although a majority of the envelopes have a diameter of 180 mμ. The edge of the envelope appears to be denser than the rest of the structure, so that one observes a membrane which varies in thickness from about 4 mμ to 5 mμ to 10 mμ. There are projections on the surface of the envelope that are about 8 mμ to 10 mμ long and that are spaced at intervals of about 5 mμ. When this structure is examined in thin-section, after permanganate fixation, the double-layered or triple-layered membrane has the appearance identical to that of the cell membrane; it also appears to have the same kind of structure as the vacuolar membrane (EPSTEIN, 1962a and b).

The function of the viral envelope is not entirely clear. Enveloped particles are more readily adsorbed to susceptible cells than are naked particles (HOLMES and WATSON, 1961) and the envelope may therefore play a role in the infectivity of the virus. This was also indicated by the experiments of SMITH (1964) in which the viral particles present in a preparation of herpes simplex virus were separated according to their buoyant density in gradients of cesium chloride. Because the presence of the envelopes will affect the buoyant density of the viral particle, the separation of enveloped and non-enveloped particles can, in principle, be accomplished by this method. The different fractions obtained from the gradient were examined with the electron microscope for the presence or absence of envelopes and were tested for virus infectivity. A strong correlation was found between the presence of envelopes and infectivity. These data imply that the viral envelope is essential for infectivity.

However, an analysis by WATSON et al. (1964) of the kinetics of formation of naked, enveloped, and infectious herpes simplex virus particles in BHK 21 cells showed that the level of infectivity exceeded that expected on the basis of the number of enveloped particles in the virus preparations. It appeared from their data that naked viral particles can also be infectious.

B. Physical-chemical Structure
1. Chemical Composition

It had been assumed for many years that the nucleic acid present in herpes simplex and pseudorabies viruses is DNA. This assumption was based primarily on indirect evidence, such as the fact that during certain stages of virus development, the intranuclear inclusions formed in cells infected with herpes simplex virus are Feulgen-positive. Since these inclusion bodies presumably contain DNA, it was concluded, therefore, that the virus also contains DNA (CROUSE et al., 1950). A few years later it was shown that infection with herpes simplex virus (NEWTON and STOKER, 1958) and with pseudorabies virus (KAPLAN and BEN-PORAT, 1959) leads to an increase in the rate of synthesis of DNA in the virus-infected cells (see below). Moreover, inhibition of the synthesis of DNA in the infected cells also inhibits the synthesis of infectious pseudorabies virus (KAPLAN and BEN-PORAT, 1961).

All these experiments provided indirect, suggestive evidence that herpes simplex and pseudorabies viruses contain DNA. However, direct meaningful analysis of the chemical composition of the viruses could be achieved only after the virus preparations had been freed of extraneous impurities. By means of improved techniques, which have become available recently, it has been possible to purify herpes simplex and pseudorabies viruses sufficiently to permit chemical analysis and to show unequivocally that these viruses contain DNA (BEN-PORAT and KAPLAN, 1962; RUSSELL, 1962a). In view of the importance of the purification of viruses in the determination of their chemical composition, it may be profitable to mention the procedures by which purification has been achieved.

Herpes simplex virus, grown in HeLa cells, was purified by the following procedure (TAVERNE and WILDY, 1959; WILDY et al., 1960; RUSSELL, 1962). The virus, separated from much of the non-viral material by differential centrifugation, was incubated with DNase and RNase and was then adsorbed to a calcium phosphate (Brushite) column in 0.2 M phosphate buffer. The virus adsorbed to the column was washed with 0.1 M phosphate buffer to remove most of the remaining impurities and was then eluted with 0.4 M phosphate buffer and dialyzed against distilled water. By this method, herpes simplex virus was purified considerably as judged by the following criteria: (1) an increase in the infectivity: protein ratio by a factor of approximately 20,000; (2) the absence of particulate matter other than the characteristic viral particles as observed in the electron microscope. It should be noted that the virus was not completely free from host material because the preparations still had some alkaline phosphatase activity and reacted in complement fixation tests with sera prepared against host cells.

When herpes simplex, purified by this method, was analyzed chemically, the virus was found to contain 70% protein, 22% phospholipid, 1.5% carbohydrate, and 6.5% DNA (RUSSELL et al., 1963). This analysis has not yet been confirmed, and whether it represents a precise estimation of the chemical composition of herpes simplex virus remains to be ascertained.

Pseudorabies virus (BEN-PORAT and KAPLAN, 1962) was first partially purified by differential centrifugation and the viral particles were then separated from extraneous impurities by means of equilibrium centrifugation of the preparation in gradients of cesium chloride (MESELSON et al., 1957). According to this method, a solution of cesium chloride is rotated for a sufficient time in an ultracentrifuge to produce a sedimentation-diffusion equilibrium.

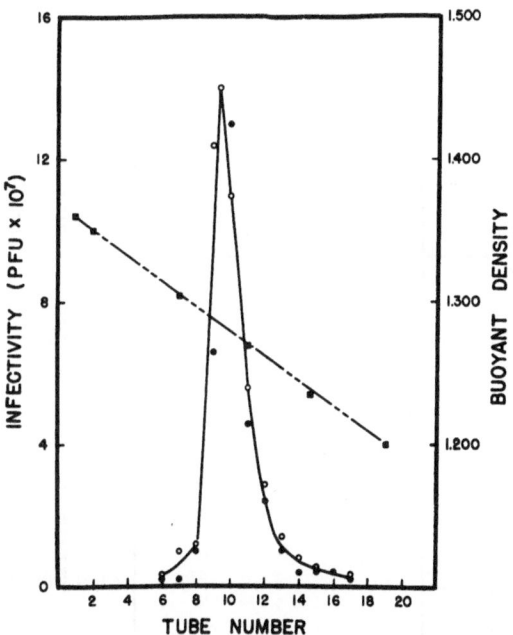

Fig. 5. The buoyant density of pseudorabies virus, as determined by isopycnic centrifugation in CsCl. The bottom of the centrifuge tube (highest density) is at the left and the top (lowest density) at the right. The circles present virus infectivity, the results of two experiments. The squares and broken line represent the density gradient (A. S. KAPLAN, unpublished results).

The cesium chloride will sediment in the direction of the field, and back-diffusion will occur as a result of the non-uniform concentration. At equilibrium, the concentration of the cesium chloride increases with distance from the center of rotation and this produces a density gradient. If virus is present in the initial solution, the virus will be forced into a unique position in the density gradient, the density of the solution at this point corresponding to the buoyant density of the virus and the virus will thereby be separated from contaminating host material. After the gradient has been established a hole is pierced in the bottom of the plastic centrifuge tube and fractions are collected drop by drop. The fractions containing the virus are identified by assaying them for infectivity or for some other parameter (radioactivity or antigenicity, for example) and the chemical composition of these fractions is then determined. An experiment illustrating this technique is given in Fig. 5. It was found that virus preparations purified by this method had a ratio of DNA to protein of approximately 1:25.

Although virus preparations purified by equilibrium sedimentation in density gradients of cesium chloride may be relatively free of cellular elements, the virus population present in the virus band may not be homogeneous with respect to its content of DNA. PFAU and MCCREA (1963) demonstrated that isopycnic centrifugation in cesium chloride fails to resolve different classes of vaccinia particles, a condition that may also be applicable to pseudorabies virus or herpes

Table 2. *Properties of the DNA of Herpes Simplex and Pseudorabies Viruses*

	Buoyant density in CsCl (gm/cm³)	Base composition[1]				Sedimentation coefficient	Molecular weight	References
		A	T	G	C			
Herpes simplex		13.9	12.9	38.0	35.2[2]			BEN-PORAT and KAPLAN (1962)
	1.727	16	16	34	34[3]	44 S	68×10^6	RUSSELL and CRAWFORD (1964)
		17.8	15.9	33.6	31.5[2]			LANDO et al. (1965)
Pseudorabies	1.732	13.2	13.5	37.0	36.3[2]		70×10^6	BEN-PORAT and KAPLAN (1962)
								KAPLAN and BEN-PORAT (1964)
	1.733	13	13	37	37[3]	44 S	68×10^6	RUSSELL and CRAWFORD (1963; 1964)
	1.732							ERIKSON and SZYBALSKI (1964)

[1] A, adenine; T, thymidine; G, guanine; C, cytosine.
[2] Determined chemically.
[3] Determined from buoyant density in density gradients of CsCl.

simplex virus and probably accounts for the low content of DNA per viral particle obtained by this method. This problem was overcome by combining treatment of the virus with fluorocarbon and centrifugation in density gradients of potassium tartrate. In this procedure, virus suspensions, buffered at pH 7.4, were homogenizad with Genetron 113 ($C_2Cl_3F_3$) at $-10°C$, centrifuged, and this homogenization repeated twice. This is a particularly sensitive step, because further treatment with Genetron caused a marked drop in infectivity. [It is of interest to note that pseudorabies virus seems to be more sensitive than herpes simplex virus to this treatment; just one treatment of this virus with Ledon 113, another fluorocarbon ($C_2F_3Cl_3$), caused a drastic drop in infectivity (IVANIČOVÁ, 1961)]. The supernatant fluids were combined and the virus concentrated with carbowax. Final purification of the herpes simplex virus preparation was achieved by centrifugation in a density gradient of potassium tartrate. This method allowed a high recovery of infectious viral particles which seemed to be relatively free of extraneous elements, as determined by electron microscopy. Using this method of purification, it was found that herpes simplex virus contains at least 10% to 11% DNA (NORCROSS et al., 1963).

The base composition of the DNA of the viruses was, in most cases, determined from their buoyant density in cesium chloride. Both herpes simplex and pseudorabies viruses contain DNA with a relatively high proportion of guanine and cytosine (Table 2). The base composition of pseudorabies virus DNA, as determined by chemical analysis, is in accord with the buoyant density in cesium chloride of the DNA (KAPLAN and BEN-PORAT, 1964).

In addition to DNA, the herpes viruses also contain protein and lipids. One strain of herpes simplex virus, HFEM, has been reported to contain a small amount (1.5%) of carbohydrate (RUSSELL et al., 1963). This finding has not yet been confirmed for other strains of herpes simplex virus or for pseudorabies virus.

Detailed chemical analyses of the viral components other than that of DNA have not been reported. It is clear, however, that while the capsid seems to be composed mainly of proteins, the envelopes of the viruses probably contain lipid, since they are rapidly disintegrated by treatment with ether.

The population of herpes simplex virus particles is not homogeneous with regard to their chemical composition. AURELIAN and WAGNER (1966) separated two groups of viral particles by rate zonal centrifugation in sucrose gradients: One type of viral particles sedimented relatively slowly and contained most of the infectivity. The other type, which was more numerous but less infectious, sedimented more rapidly. These two types of particles could not be distinguished morphologically, but could be differentiated by the following properties: The more rapidly sedimented particles appeared to be more heat labile, less readily neutralized by antiserum, and had a lower buoyant density in cesium chloride. These particles also contained three different kinds of DNA, one of them with the same buoyant density as cellular DNA, indicating that a portion of the population of these virions appeared to package cellular DNA within the viral particles.

2. Physical Characteristics of Viral Components

a) DNA

The DNA of herpes simplex virus (RUSSELL and CRAWFORD, 1963) and of pseudorabies virus (KAPLAN and BEN-PORAT, 1964) is double-stranded. This was adduced from the following evidence: (1) the mole fraction ratios of adenine to thymine and of guanine to cytosine are equal; (2) heat denaturation of the DNA of these viruses causes the increase in buoyant density, as well as in absorbance in the ultraviolet, expected for double-stranded DNA (MESELSON and STAHL, 1958; SUEOKA et al., 1959; SINSHEIMER, 1959); (3) viral DNA will react with formaldehyde only after heat denaturation, a behavior characteristic of double-stranded DNA (SINSHEIMER, 1959; STOLLAR and GROSSMAN, 1962; FREIFELDER and DAVISON, 1963). The molecular weight of the DNA of herpes simplex virus is 68×10^6 and of pseudorabies virus, 70×10^6.

b) Capsid

The capsid of herpes simplex virus appears to be composed of protein. The integrity of this structure is unaffected by treatment with ether. It is also unaffected by the following treatments: freezing and thawing in distilled water; incubation at 37°C over a wide pH range; incubation with proteases (trypsin, ficin, and papain); vibration by sonic oscillation. Although the capsids are remarkably stable and seem unaffected by these treatments, virus infectivity is decreased by a factor greater than one thousand and there is a marked increase in the proportion of empty capsids (WILDY et al., 1960).

Centrifugation in cesium chloride has a deleterious effect on the infectivity of pseudorabies virus (BEN-PORAT and KAPLAN, 1963) and it has been shown recently by SPRING and ROIZMAN (1967) that herpes simplex virus is actually disassembled by centrifugation in solutions of this salt.

Table 3. *Buoyant Density in CsCl of Herpes Simplex and Pseudorabies Viruses*

Virus	Strain	Buoyant density (gm/cm³)	References
Herpes simplex	MP	1.262	AURELIAN and WAGNER (1966)
	MP	1.260	ROIZMAN and ROANE (1961)
	mP	1.271	ROIZMAN and ROANE (1961)
	rR	1.2614	KOHLHAGE (1964)
	fR	1.2539	KOHLHAGE (1964)
	Lennette	1.254	FALKE (1965)
Pseudorabies		1.278	KAPLAN (unpublished results)

3. Buoyant Density of the Viruses

The buoyant density of pseudorabies virus was found to be 1.278 g/cm³ (KAPLAN and BEN-PORAT, unpublished results). This value is close to the buoyant density of 1.271 g/cm³ found by ROIZMAN and ROANE (1961) for the mP variant of herpes simplex virus. The buoyant densities of these viruses differ considerably from the buoyant density found for the MP variant of herpes simplex virus and a number of the other strains listed in Table 3.

The different densities of the viruses probably reflect differences in the amount of protein, lipid, or nucleic acid in the viral particles. The first two components probably have a greater effect on the buoyant density of these viruses than does the viral DNA. Thus, although the buoyant density of pseudorabies virus DNA is increased from 1.732 g/cm³ to 1.774 g/cm³ when about 80% of its thymine is replaced by 5-bromouracil, the density of the viral particles containing these two types of DNA differs by only 0.005 g/cm³ (KAPLAN et al., 1965). The buoyant density of a given particle of herpes simplex virus also appears to depend on the cell in which it is grown. Thus, the MP strain of herpes simplex virus possesses a buoyant density in cesium chloride of 1.268 g/cm³ when grown in HEp-2 cells, and a buoyant density of 1.281 g/cm³ when grown in chick embryo cells (SPEAR and ROIZMAN, 1967).

C. Antigenic Structure
1. Antigenic Relationships of the Herpes Viruses

Immunological techniques provide one of the most sensitive methods for distinguishing between one virus and another, especially closely related ones, and these techniques were used by early workers for this purpose. SABIN, in 1934, first examined the antigenic relationship between herpes simplex and pseudorabies virus by two methods — protection tests in rabbits and guinea pigs and neutralization tests in guinea pigs. He found that rabbits convalescent after an infection with herpes simplex virus succumbed to inoculation with pseudorabies virus. On the other hand, a few herpes simplex virus-immune guinea pigs, animals which are less susceptible than rabbits to pseudorabies virus, resisted a small but definitely infectious dose of pseudorabies virus; however, increasing the dose of the virus inoculum overcame this protection. Neutralization tests performed with guinea pigs as test animals suggested that, perhaps, there was some neutralization of pseudorabies virus by herpes simplex virus antisera; however, no reciprocal neutralization was obtained. These results suggested to SABIN (1934) that there may be a partial immunological relationship between pseudorabies and herpes simplex viruses. However, later investigators, using modern, more accurate methods of analysis could detect no immunological relationship between these two viruses (KAPLAN and VATTER, 1959; PLUMMER, 1964; WATSON et al. 1967). Herpes simplex virus and pseudorabies virus are also unrelated immunologically to the following members of the herpesvirus group: infectious laryngotracheitis virus, infectious bovine rhinotracheitis virus, equine herpes virus, types I and II, virus III of rabbits, varicella, and herpes zoster (FITZGERALD and HANSON, 1963; ARMSTRONG et al., 1961; PLUMMER and WATERSON, 1963; STEVENS and GROMAN, 1963; PLUMMER, 1964; ANDREWES, 1930; KAPSENBERG, 1964).

There seems to be some antigenic relationship between herpes simplex virus and B virus and also between pseudorabies virus and B virus. When B virus was first isolated from a fatal case of ascending myelitis and the virus was compared serologically with other possibly related viruses, it was found that guinea pigs which were immune to B virus came down with herpes simplex virus infection after inoculation with this virus (SABIN, 1934). However, hyperimmune serum against herpes simplex virus or B virus could neutralize small amounts of the heterologous virus when the mixture was inoculated by the subcutaneous route, but not when it was inoculated intracerebrally, indicating that there was a small but definite antigenic relationship between the two viruses. Guinea pigs convalescent from infection with B virus also resisted infection with small amounts of pseudorabies virus but succumbed when the dose was increased tenfold (SABIN, 1934). Later, BURNET et al. (1939) showed that serum obtained from mice immunized against B virus possessed considerably neutralizing activity against herpes simplex virus. Other tests by BURNET et al. (1939) indicated that not only are B virus and herpes simplex virus related antigenically, but that B virus has a broader antigenicity than herpes simplex virus.

Results similar to the ones reported by SABIN were also obtained by MELNICK and BANKER (1954), using cotton rats or neonatal mice. When these animals were inoculated intracerebrally with mixtures of B virus and serum against herpes simplex virus, neutralization of B virus was not observed, although the virus was neutralized by homologous serum. However, when rabbits were inoculated intracutaneously, serum against herpes simplex virus showed a neutralization index about 1/10 that of homologous serum. The antigenic relationship between herpes simplex virus and B virus has also been established by more recent studies (SCHNEWEIS, 1962c; PLUMMER, 1964; FALKE, 1964; BENDA, 1966; WATSON et al., 1967).

In summary, herpes simplex virus and pseudorabies virus are unrelated antigenically to each other and to most of the other members of the herpes virus group. A small but definite antigenic relationship exists, however, between herpes simplex virus and B virus and pseudorabies virus and B virus. The herpes viruses have been grouped together by virtue of many of their properties and the antigenic individuality of the various members of this group may signify divergent evolutionary pathways from a common ancestor (BURNET et al., 1939).

2. Antigenic Differences between Strains of Herpes Simplex Virus and Pseudorabies Virus

The various strains of herpes simplex virus were thought for some time to be uniform in their serological behavior, and antigenic differences between them could not be detected (BURNET et al., 1939; KILBOURNE and HORSFALL, 1951; GARABEDIAN and SYVERTON, 1955; HAYWARD, 1950). This apparent antigenic uniformity was probably due to the limited number of strains studied, as well as, perhaps, to the relative insensitivity of the serological tests employed.

However, careful analysis of a large number of strains of herpes simplex virus revealed some differences in their antigenic constitution. Thus, cross-complement fixation tests carried out by WOMACK and HUNT (1954) indicated the existence of antigenic differences between some strains of herpes simplex virus. SLAVIN and GAVETT (1946b), FLORMAN and TRADER (1947), and JAWETZ et al. (1955) also showed small differences between a number of strains of herpes simplex virus by neutralization tests and by cross-protection tests. Since this initial work, antigenic differences among various strains of herpes simplex virus have been amply reported (SHUBLADZE et al., 1960; WHEELER, 1964; SCHNEWEIS, 1962b; FALKE, 1964; HAMAR, 1964).

The degree of antigenic difference among strains of herpes simplex virus can be established by experiments in which the reduction in infectivity of a virus is measured by the plaque technique after reaction of the virus with varying dilutions of antiserum prepared against a number of strains of herpes simplex virus. Employing this technique, ROIZMAN and ROANE (1963) found that two variants of herpes simplex virus, mP and MP, are antigenically similar but not identical. ASHE and SCHERP (1963) defined the degree of antigenic difference among a large number of strains of herpes simplex virus by the kinetics of their neutralization by herpes simplex virus antisera, using plaque formation on rabbit kidney monolayer cultures to measure virus infectivity. A strain of virus can be uniquely characterized by the rate at which it is neutralized by its homologous or heterologous antiserum. The neutralization rate constant, K, is equal to $(D/t) \times 2.3 \log (V_0/V_t)$, where V_0 is the concentration of infectious virus at time 0, V_t the concentration of infectious virus at time t, and D is equal to 1/C, the dilution of the antiserum. When surviving infectious virus is plotted on a logarithmic scale against time on a linear scale, a straight line results whose slope yields the value for K. The K value of a given serum will vary for different strains of virus if these strains have different antigenic structures. It is of particular interest that ASHE and SCHERP (1963 and 1965), using this technique, found that 13 strains of herpes simplex virus isolated from recurrences of herpes labialis in four individuals could be easily distinguished antigenically. The successive isolates from the same individual frequently varied antigenically, and the serological relationships of these strains could not be correlated with their sequence or temporal proximity of recurrences or with the labial sites of the lesions. These experiments do indicate that continued multiplication of a virus, even in the same host, suffices in time to change its antigenic character. An analogous observation has been reported by HAMPAR and KEEHN (1967) who found by neutralization kinetics that in a culture persistently infected with herpes simplex virus, the virus acquires in time new antigenic determinants while still retaining the antigenic determinants of the parental virus.

The exact number of serological subgroups of herpes simplex virus is the subject of some controversy. Strains of herpes simplex virus isolated from man have been placed by SHUBLADZE et al. (1960) into three serological subgroups, as determined by neutralization tests in mice. PLUMMER (1964), on the other hand, using the tube dilution method for assay in tissue culture neutralization tests, found that herpes simplex virus fell into only two serological subgroups. In an analysis of a large number of strains of herpes simplex virus by the highly accurate method of neutralization kinetics, ASHE and SCHERP (1963) found that the majority of the strains fell into four serological groups; in addition to these four groups, the data obtained by this technique suggested the existence of two additional serogroups. Using a slightly different method of kinetic analysis, SCHNEWEIS (1962b) divided thirty strains of herpes simplex virus into only two groups: a major group of twenty six strains and a minor one of four strains.

Whatever may be the exact number of serological subgroups, it is clear that the various strains of herpes simplex virus do not constitute a homogeneous antigenic species and that variations in their antigenic makeup do exist. No such variation has been found for the strains of pseudorabies virus examined thus far.

3. Antigenic Composition

There is a limited amount of information available on the antigenic structure of herpes simplex and pseudorabies viruses. Antigenic differences between the envelope and the capsid of herpes simplex virus particles have been found. Thus, sera prepared against normal host cells agglutinated mostly enveloped herpes simplex viral particles, as observed in the electron microscope (WATSON and WILDY, 1963). On the other hand, sera prepared against herpes simplex virus agglutinated the naked capsids only, suggesting that envelopes and capsids do not share common antigens. (The apparent paradox arising from this observation and the fact that virus-specific antisera presumably neutralize the infectivity of enveloped particles remains unexplained.) That the envelope of herpes simplex virus may be related to the membrane of HeLa cells was also suggested by their structure, as observed in thin-sections in the electron microscope (EPSTEIN, 1962).

Little is known about the antigenic structure of the capsid proteins and of the proteins which are presumably present in the core. This state of affairs is not surprising, since the different protein constituents of the viral particles have not been purified and therefore specific antibody against the various proteins is not available. Individual preparations of antisera against infectious virus seem to vary in their reaction with different antigens. Thus, in one set of experiments, it was found that the viral capsid protein sub-units of pseudorabies did not have the same antigenicity as the complete viral capsid. Immediately after their synthesis, when these proteins were in a soluble state, they did not react with immune serum prepared against mature virus; they did, however, react with this antiserum, once these proteins became associated with the "naked" unenveloped viral particles which form in the nucleus of the infected cells (FUJI-WARA and KAPLAN, 1967). Thus, in this case, the antiserum used did not react with soluble viral protein. In most cases, however, serum against infectious virus does react with soluble viral proteins.

Herpes simplex virus-infected cells produce a soluble complement-fixing antigen that can be separated from the viral particles by centrifugation (HAY-WARD, 1949; WILDY and HOLDEN, 1954; SOSA-MARTINEZ and LENNETTE, 1959; SCHMIDT et al., 1960; SCHNEWEIS, 1962a; FALKE, 1965), as well as from a skin-reactive antigen (JAWETZ et al., 1951). The soluble antigen is destroyed by heating at 56°C for one hour, but can be stored for several months at 4°C with little loss of activity. The relationship of the soluble antigen to mature viral particles is not clear at present, but it is likely that at least part of this soluble antigen represents excess structural viral protein which has not become integrated into mature virions. Thus, HAMADA and KAPLAN (1965) showed that the soluble antigens of pseudorabies virus present in the cell during the earlier stages of infection became part of mature viral particles at later stages of the infective process.

4. Hemagglutination

In spite of repeated attempts, the viruses of the herpes group have not, as a rule, been found to agglutinate red blood cells. However, SHUBLADZE et al. (1960) have recently demonstrated that certain strains of herpes simplex virus will hemagglutinate goose red blood cells, provided the pH ranges between 5.2 and 6.8. Hemagglutination is prevented by specific immune sera, thus indicating that this is a specific reaction. TOKUMARU and McNAIR SCOTT (1964), on the other hand, have tested forty strains of herpes simplex virus for their ability to hemagglutinate goose erythrocytes, and in no case was hemagglutination observed. The reason for these different results is not known at present.

It is possible to obtain hemagglutination with all strains of herpes simplex virus if sheep erythrocytes treated with tannic acid are used. Herpes simplex virus will be adsorbed to these erythrocytes which can then be agglutinated by specific immune sera (SCOTT et al., 1957). The antibody involved in the hemagglutination reaction is probably identical with herpes simplex virus neutralizing antibody (FELTON and SCOTT, 1961).

D. Resistance to Physical and Chemical Agents

1. Heat

Herpes simplex virus is relatively thermolabile. According to FARNHAM and NEWTON (1959) and to SCOTT et al. (1961), this virus is inactivated at 37°C in a first order reaction. KAPLAN (1957), HOGGAN and ROIZMAN (1959), and PLUMMER and LEWIS (1965), on the other hand, have described a definite shoulder in the slope of the inactivation curve, indicating either that (1) virus clumps were present in the preparations, or (2) that cumulative temperature damage is necessary to inactivate one infectious viral particle.

SCOTT et al. (1961) found that two strains of herpes simplex virus, which produce different kinds of cytological changes, were inactivated at the same rate at 37°C; the half-life was 1.5 hours at 37°C and 3.75 hours at 30°C. The inactivation rate at 37°C was similar to that reported by POWELL (1959), who found an inactivation rate of $0.08 \log_{10}$ per hour. FARNHAM and NEWTON (1959), on the other hand, found the half-life of herpes simplex virus infectivity at 30°C, 37°C, and 44°C, to be 13, 3, and 0.4 hours, respectively. KAPLAN (1957) showed that less than 1% of herpes simplex virus infectivity survived 24 hours at 37°C; similar results were obtained by HOGGAN and ROIZMAN (1959).

Pseudorabies virus appears to be more thermostable than herpes simplex virus. For example, after 5 hours at 44°C, 28% of pseudorabies virus but only 0.014% of herpes simplex virus infectivity survived. The final slopes of the survival curves were approximately 1×10^{-2} per hour and 2×10^{-1} per hour for herpes simplex and pseudorabies virus, respectively (KAPLAN and VATTER, 1959).

2. Irradiation

Herpes simplex virus and pseudorabies virus are inactivated in an exponential manner by X-ray irradiation or ultraviolet light irradiation (POWELL, 1959; SCOTT et al., 1961; KAPLAN, 1962; PFEFFERKORN et al., 1965).

The infectivity of herpes simplex virus was reduced approximately 90% after X-radiation with a dose of about 14,000 roentgens (POWELL, 1959); the same degree of reduction in the infectivity of pseudorabies virus was obtained after γ-irradiation with a dose of about 200,000 roentgens (KAPLAN and BEN-PORAT, 1966a). About 90% of infectious pseudorabies virus was inactivated by a dose of 440 ergs/mm² of ultraviolet light irradiation (KAPLAN, 1962).

The infectivity of herpes simplex virus is destroyed in an irreversible manner by photosensitization: complexes formed in the absence of visible light between herpes simplex virus and the dyes neutral red, proflavine, or toluidine blue are extremely sensitive to inactivation by visible light (WALLIS and MELNICK, 1964).

3. Chemicals

One of the best known characteristics of the viruses of the herpes group is their extreme susceptibility to lipid solvents, such as ethyl ether (ANDREWES and HORSTMANN, 1949; KAPLAN and VATTER, 1959), sodium desoxycholate (BEDSON and GOSTLING, 1958), and chloroform (ROIZMAN and ROANE, 1963). All of these reagents affect the lipids of the virus. Nitrous acid, which reacts with nucleic acid, inactivates pseudorabies virus in a first order reaction (IVANICOVA et al., 1963). In addition to these chemicals, there are a variety of com-

pounds, ranging from metallic cations to a number of organic chemicals affecting proteins, that render herpes simplex virus noninfectious (IVANICOVA, 1961;
SERY and FURGIUELE, 1961; WHITEHOUSE et al., 1961/62; WHITE and HARRIS,
1963). Urea and sodium dodecyl sulfate also bring about a loss of infectivity
and result probably in the total destruction of the virus structure.

The herpes viruses are also inactivated by treatment with various enzymes.
Trypsin inactivates both herpes simplex virus (GRESSER and ENDERS, 1961)
and pseudorabies virus (BEN-PORAT, unpublished results, 1964). Herpes simplex virus is also inactivated by alkaline and acid phosphatases (AMOS, 1953).
These enzymes do not destroy the viral capsid and probably affect in some way
the outer envelope of the viruses, either by total destruction of the envelope or
by removal of specific sites essential for attachment to cells.

4. Virus Stability during Storage

The maintenance of stable infectious virus, one of the essential prerequisites
for any study of viruses, is greatly dependent upon the conditions of storage
(temperature and type of medium in which the virus is suspended). Herpes simplex virus suspended in medium containing serum is stable at $-70°C$ for at least
3 to 4 months or at $4°C$ for one month; storage at $-20°C$, however, reduces
infectivity more than tenfold in two weeks (STOKER and ROSS, 1958; SCHNEWEIS,
1961). Herpes simplex virus grown in chick embryos is best preserved at $-70°C$
or $-20°C$, if the virus is suspended in an equal volume of skim milk (SPECK et al.,
1951; LÉPINE et al., 1960; ANTONELLI et al., 1964). Herpes simplex virus-infected
chorioallantoic membranes suspended in glycerol or skim milk can be stored at
$-20°C$ without appreciable loss of titer; they are preserved best, however, at
$-70°C$ (ALLEN et al., 1952). The titer of pseudorabies virus is kept constant for
a long period of time at $-70°C$ when it is stored in saline (buffered with Tris
at pH 7.5) containing 1% serum albumin (KAPLAN, unpublished results).

V. Cultivation
A. Host Range

Herpes simplex virus and pseudorabies virus will multiply in a wide variety
of cells cultivated in vitro, some of which are listed in Table 4. It has been reported
that herpes simplex virus will multiply in human leukocytes in vitro, provided
the cells are supplied with phytohemagglutinin (NAHMIAS et al., 1964). This
observation may be of some clinical interest.

The different types of cells vary in their sensitivity to the viruses. Thus,
rabbit kidney cells are more sensitive to both viruses than renal cells from monkey
and from man or than chick embryo cells. Rabbit kidney cells are also equally
or more sensitive to the viruses than embryonated eggs and the brain of the mouse
(BARSKI et al., 1955).

B. Environmental Factors that Affect Virus Formation
1. Chemical Factors

Herpes simplex virus will grow in L cells maintained in a synthetic medium
in which the cells will survive but will not multiply (PELMONT and MORGAN,
1959). This maintenance medium contains all the essential amino acids but no

Table 4. *Host Cell Range*

Virus	Cells	References
Herpes simplex	Chick embryo Rabbit kidney Marmoset kidney Hamster kidney Chinese hamster Feline kidney Swine kidney HeLa KB HEp-2 Human amnion Rat lung, rabbit lung Human fibroblasts Mouse fibroblasts Rous sarcoma Tortoise kidney	STULBERG and SCHAPIRA (1953) BARSKI et al. (1955) SOSA-MARTINEZ et al. (1955) KAPLAN (1957) SCHUR and HOLMES (1965) WATSON and WILDY (1963) HAMPAR and ELLISON (1963) CRANDELL (1959) HANCOCK et al. (1959) SCHERER and SYVERTON (1954) STOKER (1959) HINZE and WALKER (1961b) KAPLAN (1957) OSTERHOUT and TAMM (1959) SZÁNTÓ (1960) ENDERS (1953) SCHERER (1953) NANKERVIS et al. (1959) FAUCONNIER (1963)
Pseudorabies	Mouse fibroblasts HeLa Rabbit kidney Swine kidney Lamb kidney Dog kidney Monkey kidney Chick embryo	SCHERER (1953) SCHERER and SYVERTON (1954) KAPLAN and VATTER (1959) SINGH (1962) McFERRAN and DOW (1962) CECCARELLI and DEL MAZZA (1958) AURELIAN and ROIZMAN (1964) VON KERÉKJÁRTÓ and RHODE (1957) ALBRECHT et al. (1963) BÉLÁDI and IVANOVICS (1954) CSEREY-PECHANY et al. (1951)

serum, the latter being essential for cell division. However, virus is not synthesized if any one of the following amino acids is omitted: phenylalanine, tryptophan, arginine, threonine, leucine, valine and histidine. On the other hand, omission of isoleucine, lysine, alanine, and glycine has no effect on the growth of herpes simplex virus in L cells. The replication of herpes simplex virus in human cells requires arginine particularly (TANKERSLEY, 1964; SHARON, 1966; JENEY et al., 1967), as well as glutamine and glucose (LEWIS and SCOTT, 1962).

If cells maintained in a simple salt solution, in which the virus cannot grow, are infected, the virus can survive in the absence of growth-requiring nutrients for several days and will start multiplying when complete medium is added (PELMONT and MORGAN, 1959). It has not been established whether the virus survives under these conditions in a coated or uncoated form.

2. Physical Factors
a) Radiation of Host Cell

The capacity of rabbit kidney cells to synthesize herpes simplex virus is highly resistant to X-ray irradiation. For example, cells irradiated with 10,000 roentgens and infected within one or two days produced the same amount of virus as un-irradiated cells. Virus also multiplied in cells irradiated with a dose as high as 40,000 roentgens. In this case, however, the yield was reduced to about 30% of that normally obtained from unirradiated cells (KAPLAN, 1957). Similar results have been reported for herpes simplex virus and X-ray irradiated L cells (POWELL, 1959).

The capacity of ERK cells to support the growth of pseudorabies virus is also greatly resistant to the action of ultraviolet light irradiation. Thus, after a dose of 660 ergs/mm², practically no loss of the capacity of the cells to form infective centers was observed; however, this dose of ultraviolet light irradiation reduced the ability of the cell population to form colonies by about 99% (KAPLAN, 1962). Because the reproductive capacity of mammalian cells is lost much more readily than their ability to produce virus, these results indicate that the host cell components affected by irradiation are not required for virus synthesis.

b) Temperature

The temperature at which infected cells are incubated plays a decisive role in the development of the herpes viruses. As in the case of most virus-cell systems, the optimal temperature range for the production of infectious herpes simplex and pseudorabies viruses is a resultant of two forces — the temperature of incubation conducive to maximal virus replication and the temperature of incubation conducive to minimal inactivation of virus infectivity. The optimal temperature for production of herpes simplex and pseudorabies viruses ranges between 35°C and 37°C, a conclusion based on the following studies.

In cultures of fragments of chick embryos, the maximal concentration of infectious virus was demonstrated when infected cultures were incubated at 35°C; infectious virus could not be detected if the cultures were incubated at 40°C (THOMPSON and COATES, 1942). Little or no virus was produced by infected HeLa cells incubated for three days at 20.5°C to 27.7°C; the greatest amount of infectious virus was recovered when the cultures were incubated at 35°C (WHEELER, 1958). FARNHAM and NEWTON (1959) showed that the latent period of herpes simplex virus in HeLa cells was extended when the infected cells were incubated at 30°C rather than at 37°C. The rate of formation of intracellular virus also was slower at 30°C than at 37°C. However, the rate of extracellular accumulation of infectious virus was not greatly affected by this difference in temperature and the yield of infectious virus after 24 hours of incubation at these temperatures was approximately the same. If, however, incubation was continued beyond 24 hours, the best yields were obtained at 31°C to 33°C; at 40.5°C very little infectious virus was detected and the final yield at this temperature was less than 0.05 pock-forming units per cell. Similar results have been reported by HOGGAN and ROIZMAN (1959a).

It is of interest to note, in this connection, that mice are more resistant to infection with herpes simplex virus when they are kept at 37°C than at 24°C. Mice maintained at an external temperature of 37°C have a rectal temperature of about 40°C, whereas mice maintained at 24°C have a rectal temperature of about 37°C (SCHMIDT and RASMUSSEN, 1960a). The lower mortality of the mice at the higher temperature could be attributed to a lower level of infectious virus present in the brains of the animals held in an environmental temperature of 37°C. These observations have important implications with respect to the role of fever in viral diseases.

C. Virus Growth Cycle

As in all interactions between viruses and their susceptible host cells, the growth cycle of herpes simplex and pseudorabies viruses may be divided into several distinct phases. In the first phase, *adsorption*, virus attaches to susceptible cells, provided proper conditions prevail; this phase is followed by *penetration* of the infectious viral particle into the interior of the cell. The protein coat of the viral

particle is removed and this un-coating of the viral particle signals the start of the *eclipse* phase, which may be defined as that stage of the virus growth cycle during which infectious virus cannot be detected within the infected cells. This phase comes to an end with the produc-tion of the first intracellular infec-tious viral particle. The period of virus eclipse constitutes the first part of the *latent period* which ends upon release of the first infectious viral particle to the surrounding me-dium. The final phase of the infective process is called the period of "*expo-nential*" *virus increase*, during which most of the mature virions are pro-duced; the end of this period marks the end of the virus growth cycle.

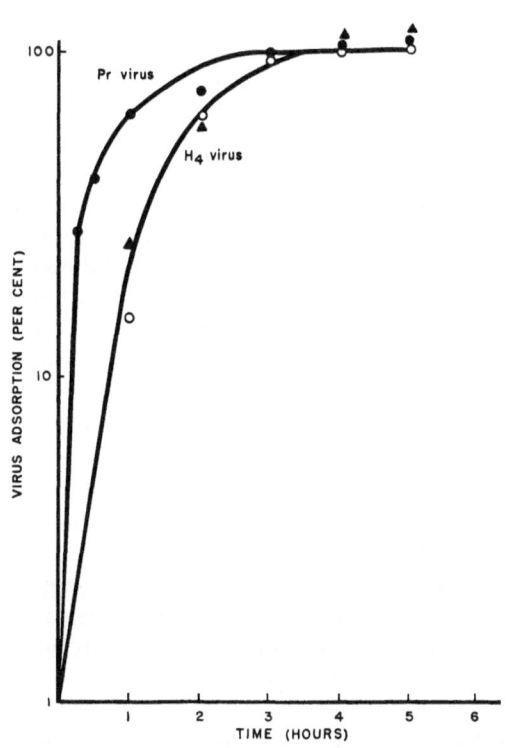

1. Adsorption

The rate of adsorption of herpes simplex virus and pseudorabies virus to susceptible cells appears to be little affected by temperature or by cyanide (FARNHAM and NEWTON, 1959; KAPLAN, 1962). Attachment of herpes simplex virus to cells re-

Fig. 6. The adsorption of herpes simplex and pseudo-rabies viruses to monolayers of rabbit kidney cells. Closed circles, pseudorabies virus; triangles and open circles, herpes simplex virus. The adsorption curve for herpes simplex virus represents the results of two experiments. From A. S. KAPLAN and A. E. VATTER, Virology 7, 394 (1959).

quires the presence of electrolytes in the adsorption medium, particularly calcium and magnesium (FARNHAM and NEWTON, 1959). Thus, as in the case of bacterio-phage and other viruses, adsorption of pseudorabies and herpes simplex viruses is probably an electrostatic process involving the ionic groups on the surfaces of the viruses and their host cells.

The rate of adsorption of the two viruses is dependent, as expected, upon the relative concentrations of virus and cells. For example, FARNHAM (1958) found that when the same amount of virus was added to cultures in volumes of

1 ml, 0.5 ml or 0.1 ml, the relative number of plaques obtained was 1, 1.5 and 1.7, respectively. The adsorption rate also seems to vary with different virus strains and cells (Fig. 6). The adsorption of the H 4 strain of herpes simplex virus to mono-layers of rabbit kidney cells (KAPLAN, 1957) and the HFEM strain to monolayers of chick embryo cells (WATERSON, 1958) was relatively slow, with approximately 50% of the virus being adsorbed in 90 minutes. A much faster rate was found for the adsorption of the HFEM and Nash strains of herpes simplex virus to HeLa cells (FARNHAM, 1958; WATKINS, 1960); at least 50% of the virus was adsorbed within fifteen minutes. The adsorption of pseudorabies virus to rabbit kidney cells was also relatively rapid (50% in 30 minutes) (KAPLAN and VATTER, 1959); how-ever, the rate of adsorption of pseudorabies virus to chick embryo cells was much lower (BÉLÁDI, 1962).

The addition of agar to monolayers effectively arrests the process of virus adsorption (YOUNGNER, 1956; KAPLAN, 1957). This effect may be due to the fact that agar contains sulfated polysaccharides that inhibit the attachment of herpes viruses to the host cells (see below).

The adsorption of herpes simplex virus has been observed directly with the electron microscope (HOLMES and WATSON, 1963; EPSTEIN et al., 1964). Attach-ment of the virus appeared to be rapid and by 45 minutes at 36°C at least 90% of the input viral particles appeared to have attached to the cell surface; fewer particles appeared to adsorb at 0°C. Enveloped particles adsorbed more readily than naked particles to baby hamster cells and to HeLa cells.

2. Penetration

The movement of viral particles from the surface to the interior of the cells can be followed, because cell-adsorbed virus remains sensitive to the action of specific antiserum, but once the virus has penetrated into the cells, it becomes inaccessible to antiserum. The time required for the penetration of adsorbed virus can thus be measured by adding virus-specific antiserum at various times after adsorption. Using this technique, FARNHAM and NEWTON (1959) found that by four hours after inoculation practically all the adsorbed herpes simplex virus (HFEM strain) had penetrated into HeLa cells incubated at 37°C; however, only about 30% and less than 19% of the adsorbed virus was no longer neutralized by the antiserum when the cells were incubated at 30°C and 4°C, respectively. HUANG and WAGNER (1964) studied the rate of penetration of herpes simplex virus by the technique described above, as well as by another more reliable method which is based on the fact that free or attached virus is sensitive to acid (pH 3), while virus that has penetrated into the cell is not. These authors found also that penetration of the virus into the cell is temperature dependent, and whereas at 25°C twenty minutes were required before 90% of the attached virus had pene-trated, at 37°C only 10 minutes were required. Furthermore, at 4°C less than 1% of the virus had penetrated into the cell after one hour, as determined by acid sensitivity test. (Under the same conditions, 15% of the virus could not be neu-tralized by antibody, indicating that virus which is attached to the cell membrane is more resistant than free virus to neutralization by antibody and that therefore resistance to antiserum is not a reliable criterion for virus pene-tration.)

Thus, in contrast to adsorption, the process of virus penetration into the cells is greatly dependent upon temperature, indicating that an enzyme may be involved in this process. That energy is required for the penetration of adsorbed virus is shown by the fact that whereas cyanide did not prevent the adsorption of pseudorabies virus, it did prevent the penetration of the virus into the cell; this inhibition could be reversed by washing out the cyanide (KAPLAN, 1962).

Penetration of the viral particles has been studied also with the electron microscope (HOLMES and WATSON, 1963; EPSTEIN et al., 1964). These direct observations confirmed the results obtained by biological techniques; that is, in contrast to virus attachment, virus penetration into the cells is a temperature-dependent process. The attached viral particles appeared to enter into the cells by being surrounded by surface invaginations and by phagocytosis into cytoplasmic vacuoles. The envelopes seemed to be stripped from viral particles in these vacuoles; naked capsids could be seen subsequently in the cytoplasm. However, the precise nature of the events that occur after penetration are as yet unknown; thus, the movement of the particles from the vacuoles to the cytoplasm has not been observed.

Hormones appear to affect the adsorption and penetration of herpes simplex virus. Treatment of cells with thyroid extract prior to infection increased the rate of adsorption of virus to the cells; penetration of adsorbed virus into hormone-treated cells was also more rapid than into untreated cells. Parathyroid had an opposite effect (ROIZMAN, 1962). The reason for these hormonal effects is obscure.

3. Eclipse Period

Many of the events essential to the synthesis of viruses take place during the eclipse phase when infectious virus cannot be detected within the infected cells. Some of the enzymes which are induced by infection and which are probably necessary for the formation of viral components make their first appearance at this time. During this period, it appears that a critical mass of viral DNA and viral structural protein must accumulate before these components can be assembled into the first mature viral particle, an event that signals the end of the eclipse period. Hence, the eclipse period may be defined as that phase of the growth cycle when the cell prepares itself for the synthesis of viral particles.

The eclipse phase in herpes virus-infected cells is sometimes difficult to demonstrate, because of the problem of the residual virus inoculum. Thus, for example, the length of the eclipse period will seem to differ depending upon whether the experiments are performed in monolayer cultures or in cell suspensions. This is probably so, because the end of the latent period becomes evident only by a rise in titer great enough to exceed the residual, unadsorbed virus which is difficult to remove by washing from monolayer cultures but which is more readily eliminated from cell suspensions. (The use of cell suspensions presents the added experimental advantage that the cells may be diluted sufficiently so that there is only a slight probability of readsorption of released virus.) The problem of unadsorbed virus can, however, be overcome if the suspended, virus-infected cells are washed sufficiently (KAPLAN, 1957) or if the residual virus is eliminated by mild ultraviolet light irradiation, followed by washing, a procedure that does not affect the ability of the cells to produce virus (YOSHINO et al., 1960). Using these proce-

dures, the eclipse phase of herpes simplex virus in rabbit kidney cells was found
to be 4 hours and in the ectodermal cells of the chorioallantoic membrane of de-
embryonated eggs, 10 to 11 hours. Thus, the length of the eclipse period depends
on the cell system used and probably also upon the virus strain. Table 5 summarizes
the data for a few virus-cell systems.

The length of the eclipse period is probably also dependent upon the multiplicity of infection (see Fig. 7). Thus, KAPLAN (1957) showed that the latent
period with a low virus input was 7 hours, while with a high virus input it was
5 hours, a shift of 2 hours. This shift probably reflects a difference in the length
of the eclipse period and suggests that more than one viral particle may participate
in the initiation of the infective process.

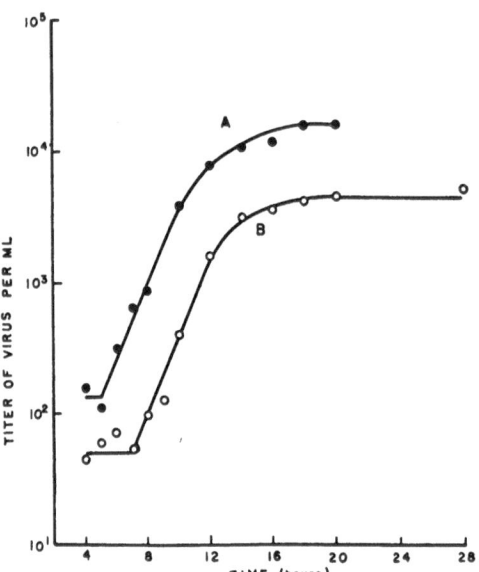

Fig. 7. The growth curve of herpes simplex virus in suspensions of rabbit kidney cells. Curve A, virus:cell ratio
of 64; curve B, virus:cell ratio of 1.6. From A. S.
KAPLAN, Virology 4, 435.(1957).

The eclipse phase of a virus may
also be shortened if cells are first
infected with a different strain of
the same virus. Thus, when HEp-2
cells were infected with the mP
strain of herpes simplex virus and
superinfected three hours later with
the MP strain of the virus, the dura-
tion of the eclipse phase normally
observed for MP virus was considerably reduced. These results indicate that substances are formed
during the eclipse phase that are
necessary for virus synthesis and
that may be used interchangeably
for the formation of either mP or
MP strains (ROIZMAN, 1963).

An eclipse period of viral particles at the beginning of the viral
growth cycle can also be detected
by electron microscopy, since during
this period the infecting viral particles   presumably   disintegrate.
Virus eclipse probably starts by the removal of the outer envelope of the viral
particle, since naked particles are much less infectious than the enveloped particles
(SMITH, 1964; HOLMES and WATSON, 1963). This process appears to take place in
phagocytic vacuoles and occurs soon after the ingestion of the viral particles.
Since enveloped particles are seen only rarely within the cytoplasm of infected
cells, this first step in the eclipse phase is readily recognizable by electron microscopy (EPSTEIN, 1964). However, the dissolution of the viral capsid is difficult
to observe, probably because to observe the viral particles within the cells, high
multiplicities of infection must be used Furthermore, the ratio of PFU:viral
particles is low and most of the particles may remain inert and behave in a
different manner from the infectious particles. Thus, RUSSELL et al. (1964) examined the actual number of viral particles within the infected cells and did not
observe their "eclipse".

HOLMES and WATSON (1963), however, studying by the same method the events that occur during the growth cycle of herpes simplex virus in baby hamster kidney cells found that most, but not all, of the viral particles had disappeared by 3 hours after the virus had penetrated into the cells. In the same experiment, an increase in the number of particles per cell was apparent 4 hours after penetration. These electron microscopic observations are in accord with the dynamics of virus growth, because the formation of infectious viral particles can first be detected in baby hamster kidney cells at about this time.

4. Latent Period

Whereas, as mentioned above, the end of the eclipse period occurs when the first infectious viral particle is formed by the infected cell, the end of the latent period is signalled by the release of the first infectious viral particle from the cell to the surrounding medium. The lengths of the latent period in several virus-cell systems are given in Table 5.

The time that elapses between the formation of the viral particles and their release from the cells can be estimated by following the rate of intracellular development and extracellular accumulation of the viral particles. The virus release time can be calculated by the following equation derived by RUBIN et al. (1955): $1/k = (t_2 - t_1)/r\ (\ln c_2 - \ln c_1)$, where $1/k$ = average release time; r = the constant ratio of extracellular virus to intracellular virus at any time during the exponential rise; t_1, t_2 = two selected times during the exponential rise; $\ln c_1, \ln c_2$ = natural logarithms of the concentra-

Table 5. *Multiplication of Herpes Simplex and Pseudorabies Viruses*

Virus	Cells	Phase of growth cycle			Virus yield (PFU/cell)	References
		Eclipse	Latent	Exponential increase		
		Hours				
Herpes simplex H 4 strain	Rabbit kidney monolayers	5	8	10	300	KAPLAN (1957)
Herpes simplex HFEM strain	HeLa monolayers	12	16	15		STOKER and ROSS (1958)
Herpes simplex H 4 strain	Rabbit kidney suspension	4	5—7	7	100—300	KAPLAN (1957)
Herpes simplex HRE strain	L suspension	5	8.5	4—5		POWELL (1959)
Pseudorabies	Rabbit kidney suspension	3	5	5	1,000	KAPLAN and VATTER (1959)
Pseudorabies	Rabbit kidney monolayers		5	5	820	KAPLAN and VATTER (1959)
Pseudorabies	Monkey kidney monolayers		12	12		VON KERÉKJÁRTÓ and ROHDE (1957)

tions of extracelluar virus at times t_1 and t_2. By means of this equation, it was calculated that for dilute suspensions of herpes simplex virus-infected rabbit kidney cells
(KAPLAN, 1957) the release time was 2.3 to 3.5 hours. In L cells infected with the
HRE strain of herpes simplex virus the release time was calculated to be 30 to
40 minutes (POWELL, 1959).

Cells in the form of monolayers or in suspension are mass cultures in which
the end of the latent period is signalled by a rise in the plaque count above that
of the base line. Thus, it is possible to establish by this method a minimal latent
period. However, since the infective process may not be synchronized, some of
the cells may not release virus until a later time. A variation in the length of the
latent period of individual cells becomes evident when each infected cell is incubated in isolated drops of nutrient medium and the latent period in each cell is
determined. In HeLa cells infected with herpes simplex virus, a variation between
16 and 26 hours was obtained (WILDY et al., 1959). In individual rabbit kidney
cells, the latent period of pseudorabies virus ranged from 6 to 10 hours (REISSIG
and KAPLAN, 1960). In both cases the shortest latent period observed in single
cells was longer than the minimum latent period determined in mass culture
(see Table 5). A longer latent period in single cells as compared to mass cultures
has also been described for monkey kidney cells infected with poliovirus (LWOFF
et al., 1955). In this case, it was suggested that the longer latent period in single
cells may have been due to a selection of late releasers; the cells in the monolayers had been infected before being isolated as single cells and only those cells
in the early phase of the infective process still able to attach to the glass were
studied. In the experiments with pseudorabies virus, selection of late releasers
could be ruled out since the single cells were infected after their attachment
to the glass. The longer latent periods in single cells are probably, therefore,
a reflection of different, probably unfavorable, experimental conditions.

The variation in time of virus release from the individual cells may be ascribed to an asynchrony in the initiation of virus synthesis in individual cells,
as observed with influenza virus (CAIRNS, 1957), or, as shown for poliovirus by
HOWES (1959), it may be ascribed to an asynchrony in the maturation of virus
in the different cells. The delay in the production of virus by some cells appears
to be determined by each virus-cell encounter and does not appear to depend
upon the state of individual cells, because an increase in the number of viral
particles infecting each cell synchronizes the infective process considerably.
The reasons for the variation in the length of the latent period of the singly
infected individual cells are, however, not knqwn at the present time.

5. Period of "Exponential" Virus Increase and Virus Release

During the period of exponential virus increase, the synthesis of virus precursor
material continues and it is during this phase of the virus growth cycle that
most of the infectious, mature viral particles are assembled from the accumu-
lating virus precursor materials and are released into the surrounding medium.

The growth of a virus depends not only upon the characteristics of the virus
itself, but also upon the type of cells infected, and the type of culture (monolayer, cell suspension, or single cell) being studied. The lengths of the periods of
exponential virus increase of some of the herpes simplex and pseudorabies virus
cell systems are given in Table 5.

The kinetics of virus synthesis appear to be exponential, but the precise mean-
ing of this observation is not clear. Presumably, the underlying cause of an exponential increase in mature virus would be the exponential synthesis of a limiting component necessary for virus formation. DNA is the only component known
to duplicate exponentially; however, DNA is not responsible for the apparent
logarithmic increase of mature virus and is not the limiting factor in virus maturation (KAPLAN, 1962; KAPLAN and BEN-PORAT, 1966b). Thus, the observed
kinetics may only be a reflection of increasing level of activities of some enzymes
or of increasing rates of synthesis of a precursor necessary for the process of virus
maturation.

The final yield of virus produced by infected cells depends upon a number of
factors, such as the type of cell infected, the thermostability of the virus, the
temperature of incubation, and whether mass cultures or single cells are studied.
Thus, rabbit kidney cells in the form of monolayer cultures yielded approximately
300 PFU per cell of herpes simplex virus. On the other hand, individual HeLa
cells yielded, on the average, about 8 pock-forming units per cell, with a considerable scatter from cell to cell (WILDY et al., 1959). The lower yields and the large
variation in PFU produced by single cells as compared with mass cultures were
also obtained with pseudorabies virus-infected cells. Suspensions of rabbit kidney cells yielded about 1,000 PFU per cell (KAPLAN and VATTER, 1959), while
the yield from individual rabbit kidney cells varied from 63 PFU to 500 PFU
per cell (REISSIG and KAPLAN, 1960). The lower yields from single cells probably
reflect the unfavorable cultural conditions as compared to those of mass cultures.

Not all the particles produced by the cells are infectious. It has been found
that the ratio of viral particles observed in the electron microscope to infective
units is 10, even under the best conditions (WATSON et al., 1963).

Herpes simplex virus may be released from cells not as individual viral particles but in the form of aggregates. Neither simple dilution nor treatment of the
virus with nucleases has any effect on the aggregates and does not increase the
virus titer. Furthermore, because the linear relationship found between virus
concentration and the number of plaques is not affected by virus dilution, the
aggregated virus apparently is not easily disaggregated (KAPLAN, 1957). The
titer of virus released from rabbit kidney cells can be increased by freezing
and thawing, and, even more effectively, by sonic oscillation, procedures which
disaggregate the clumps of virus. The increase in the titer of herpes simplex virus
after sonic oscillation has been confirmed recently in another system (SMITH, 1963).

6. Indirect Methods of Analysis of the Infective Process

Radiation has been a useful tool for probing the intracellular events that
occur during the latent period of virus development. The studies with ultraviolet light and X-ray irradiation on the interaction of animal viruses and their
host cells have been modeled after the experiments performed with bacteriophage. Two basic types of approach to this question have been used: one is the
so-called Luria-Latarjet experiment (LURIA and LATARJET, 1947) in which,
at various times after infection, the virus-cell complexes are irradiated by ultraviolet light or X-rays; the second is the photoreactivation by visible light of
ultraviolet light-irradiated virus in infected cells (DULBECCO, 1950).

Herpes simplex virus-cell complexes have been analyzed by a Luria-Latarjet type of experiment with X-rays and ultraviolet light (POWELL, 1959), and pseudo-rabies virus-cell complexes with ultraviolet light (KAPLAN, 1962). As in the case of the T-even bacteriophages and their host bacteria, the capacity of the host cells to support virus growth was found to be much more resistant to ultraviolet light irradiation than the survival of free virus. When the virus-cell complexes were irradiated at various times after infection, a family of survival curves of de-creasing slopes, which were of the single-hit type, were observed. This increased resistance of the virus-cell complexes in time after infection to radiation was dependent upon DNA synthesis, suggesting that multiplicity reactivation was the basis for the progressive stabilization of the complexes to ultraviolet light irradiation damage.

The lethal damage to the viral genome caused by irradiation with ultra-violet light can be reversed in virus-infected cells but not in free virus by ex-posure to light of longer wave length (DULBECCO, 1955; JAGGER, 1958). Ir-radiation causes the formation of thymine dimers from adjacent thymine bases on a DNA chain (SETLOW and SETLOW, 1962; WACKER et al., 1960); visible light activates an enzyme that repairs the damage (RUPERT et al., 1958; RUPERT, 1962a, b).

Pseudorabies and herpes simplex virus-infected cell complexes, inactivated by irradiation with ultraviolet light at 260 mμ, could, under certain conditions, be photo-reactivated by irradiation with visible light in the range of 300 to 420 mμ (PFEFFERKORN et al., 1965; PFEFFERKORN et al., 1966). As in the case of bacteriophage T2, photoreactivation occurred only in the infected cells, not with free virus. Little photoreactivation occurred for the first twenty minutes after adsorption of these viruses to the cells; thereafter, photoreactivation in-creased and reached a maximum at about 100 minutes after adsorption. These results suggest that this period represents the time required for the viral particle to be uncoated.

D. Plaque Formation

Plaque formation is based on the principle that an infectious virus which comes in contact with a susceptible cell will multiply within this cell and destroy it. The newly-formed viral particles will then be released and will spread to other cells in the culture. If this process is restricted to the neighboring cells, a recogniz-able focus of destroyed cells will be formed for every infectious viral particle that has infected a cell of the monolayer culture. The advantages of the plaque tech-nique for the assay of viruses rest on its relative accuracy, the rapidity of plaque formation, and economy.

Because the herpes viruses cause destruction of the cells in which they multiply, it was to be expected that suitable systems would be found for the production of virus plaques. Utilizing the finding by ANDREWES (1930) that herpes simplex virus will multiply in cells even when immune serum is present in the culture medium, BLACK and MELNICK (1955) showed that plaques of herpes-B virus will form in monolayer cultures of monkey kidney cells incubated with specific anti-serum. The antiserum prevents virus released into the medium from infect-ing cells at random but does not prevent the passage of infectious virus from cell to neighboring cell, thus permitting recognizable plaques to be formed.

The random distribution of released virus and the consequent infection of cells beyond the initial focus may also be eliminated by the use of agar instead of immune serum. Monolayer cultures of rabbit kidney cells on which agar has been laid after adsorption of herpes simplex virus will form recognizable plaques (KAPLAN, 1957). Agar eliminates the convection of viral particles that occurs in a liquid overlay but does not prevent the diffusion of virus from one cell to another. If a vital dye, such as neutral red, is added to the agar, plaques will appear as white areas against a red background (dead cells do not take up this dye). There is a linear relationship between the concentration of virus and the number of plaques that are formed, indicating that only one infectious herpes simplex virus particle is necessary to give rise to one plaque (KAPLAN, 1957; FARNHAM, 1958).

The size of the plaques formed varies according to the strain of virus and the type of cell. In rabbit kidney cells herpes simplex virus plaques begin to appear on the second day but do not reach their maximum size and number until about 4 to 6 days of incubation. By the fourth day, most of the plaques reach a size of about 1 mm to 2 mm in diameter and do not continue to increase in size. Plaques of about the same size appear in monolayer cultures of chick embryo fibroblasts (DE MAYER and SCHONNE, 1964), but somewhat smaller plaques are formed on HeLa cells (FARNHAM, 1958) and somewhat larger plaques on human amnion cells (OSTERHOUT and TAMM, 1959).

The efficiency of plaque formation with herpes simplex is relatively low in agar. A sulfated polysaccharide present in agar is responsible for the inhibition of virus growth (TAKEMOTO and FABISCH, 1964). [Other polyanions, such as the synthetic polysaccharide, sodium dextran sulfate, and heparin also inhibit herpes simplex virus growth by preventing the attachment of the virus to the cells (VAHERI and CANTELL, 1963; NAHMIAS et al., 1964)]. This inhibition can be overcome if a polycation, such protamine sulfate, is added to the agar; a significantly greater number of plaques is then observed (TYTELL and NEUMAN, 1963). The efficiency of plating is increased even further (about tenfold) and the plaques are larger if, instead of agar, the overlay consists of methyl cellulose (TYTELL and NEUMAN, 1963) or starch gel (DE MAYER and SCHONNE, 1964).

As a variation of these techniques, cells may be infected in suspension and then plated in petri dishes. The noninfected cells grow to form monolayers in which the infected cells form foci of infection. Instead of agar, secondary plaque formation is prevented by the addition of virus-specific antisera to the fluid overlay medium. After a few days of incubation, the culture fluids are removed, the undestroyed, noninfected cells are fixed with formalin and stained and the plaques are counted using a hand lens (RUSSELL, 1962 b).

That pseudorabies virus could also form plaques was first demonstrated with monolayer cultures which were overlaid with a film of chicken plasma and chicken embryonic extract (BÉLÁDI and SZÖLLÖSY, 1955). It is more convenient, however, to use agar rather than a plasma clot and various types of monolayer cultures have been found suitable for this purpose, including cultures of monkey kidney cells (YOUNGNER, 1956; VON KERÉKJÁRTO and ROHDE, 1957), rabbit kidney cells (KAPLAN and VATTER, 1959), and bovine and pig kidney cells (SINGH, 1962). In general, plaques of pseudorabies virus appear sooner and are larger than the plaques formed by herpes simplex virus.

VI. Cytopathogenicity

Infection with virulent viruses engenders profound changes in their host cells, causing them to undergo degeneration and, eventually, death. The members of the herpes group of viruses are of this type, and infection with pseudorabies virus and herpes simplex virus results, in general, in degenerative changes in and the final killing of susceptible cells.

One of the first effects of virus infection is the inhibition of mitosis. Thus, infection of a HeLa cell with one infectious viral particle suffices to inhibit mitosis in this cell. It is likely that the inhibition of mitosis is a rapid event, occurring certainly within a short period of time after virus attachment (STOKER and NEWTON, 1959). Mitosis in rabbit kidney cells is also prevented by infection with pseudorabies virus (REISSIG and KAPLAN, 1960).

After infection of susceptible cells and before their death, the cells undergo a series of cytopathic alterations that are characteristic of the infecting virus and that are most likely related to the mode of intracellular replication of the virus. The most striking cytological feature of infection with herpes simplex and pseudorabies viruses is the formation of intranuclear inclusions. However, other general cytopathological changes also occur. In this section, these latter changes in cells infected with pseudorabies virus and herpes simplex virus will be first examined; this will be followed by a description of the development of the intranuclear inclusion.

A. Gross Cytopathology

In general, the characteristic changes in cells infected with herpes simplex or pseudorabies viruses are of two types: (1) the infected cells may form syncytia, also known as polykaryocytes, which consist of large multinucleated cells, or (2) they may become rounded, frequently ballooned, with an occasional formation of small giant cells. These two types of cellular degeneration were described more than 40 years ago by LAUDA and REZEK (1926). Since that time there have been many descriptions of the two kinds of cytopathologic changes in virus-infected cells isolated from human patients (BLANK et al., 1951; WOMACK and RANDALL, 1953) and in infected cells cultivated in vitro (SCHERER, 1953; STULBERG and SCHAPIRA, 1953; ENDERS, 1953; SCHERER and SYVERTON, 1954; KAPLAN and VATTER, 1959; SCOTT and McLEOD, 1959; HOGGAN and ROIZMAN, 1959).

The formation of syncytia starts in ill-defined loci scattered throughout the virus-infected monolayer cultures. Among the normal cells, one may see groups of swollen cells the contiguous membranes of which appear to lyse and disappear. The initial syncytial mass may at first be limited by cells that appear to be normal; these cells, which may be noninfected, fuse in due time with their infected neighbors. This process continues with the eventual fusion of the cells into larger and larger syncytial masses. The nuclei appear to collect in the center of the syncytium and are surrounded by cytoplasm; many of the nuclei at this point contain inclusion bodies. However, ROIZMAN (1961) found that the syncytia formed by herpes simplex virus-infected cells may contain nuclei in prophase and mitotic figures resembling chromosomes at metaphase.

The second type of cellular degeneration, as observed in cell culture, starts with cytoplasmic granulation, followed by the conversion of the cells into a rounded refractile state, frequently called balloon cells. In time, these rounded cells increase in number within discrete foci until there is a piled up mass of cells. Finally, piles of cells appear like bunches of grapes and eventually lysis occurs. However, sometimes the cells appear clumped together instead of piling up. It was at first thought that this cytopathological expression is due to another virus variant (GRAY et al., 1958). However, SCOTT and McLEOD (1959) showed that the kind of effect one observes — clumping or piling up — is not the result of a difference in the infecting virus, but is due to the character of the mono-layer or age of the cells.

It is not essential that mature virus be formed for the development of cytopathic changes. REISSIG and KAPLAN (1962) have observed characteristic cytopathic changes in monolayer cultures of rabbit kidney cells in which the synthesis of mature pseudorabies virus was inhibited by 5-fluorouracil or Mito-mycin-C. These results suggest that the cytologic changes resulting from infection of the cells with pseudorabies virus are events independent of the formation of infectious virus.

The kind of effect (rounding or syncytia formation) one observes (see Fig. 8) is dependent upon the genetic constitution of the infecting virus. Thus, variants which produce one or the other type of cellular degeneration have been repeatedly isolated (SCOTT and McLEOD, 1959; NII and KAMAHORA, 1961; HOGGAN and ROIZMAN, 1959b; MUNK and DONNER, 1963; WHEELER, 1964; KOHLHAGE and SCHIEFERSTEIN, 1965). A third variant which is reported to cause the cells to become fusiform has also been isolated (NII, 1961).

Variants of the first two types have been well characterized by HOGGAN and ROIZMAN (1959b) who described a microplaque variant which forms small clumps of rounded cells and a macroplaque variant which produces giant multi-nucleated cells that reach diameters of 4 mm to 5 mm. Although these vari-ants breed true regardless of the type of cell they infect, the phenotypic ex-pression of the cytopathic changes may be influenced by the external environ-ment.

Variants of pseudorabies virus producing different kinds of cytopathic effects have also been formed. TOKUMARU (1957) has isolated by the limit dilution tech-nique two strains of this virus that cause either rounding of the infected cells or giant cell formation.

The type of cell infected also seems to affect the cytopathology of the virus-cell complex. The same virus isolates will produce different kinds of cytopathic effects depending on the cell culture they infect.

Thus, in addition to the genotype of the infecting virus, its phenotypic expres-sion, as modified by the host cells, will also influence the type of cytopathic effect produced (MUNK and DONNER, 1963; KOHLHAGE and SCHIEFERSTEIN, 1965).

Despite differences in cytopathic changes induced by variants of the virus, most of their other biological properties seem, in general, to be identical. How-ever, the giant cell-forming variant can be separated from the cell-rounding variant by centrifugation in density gradients of cesium chloride and on columns of ECTEOLA (ROIZMAN and ROANE, 1961; KOHLHAGE, 1964). Moreover, small antigenic differences between these two variants have been found (ROIZMAN and ROANE, 1963).

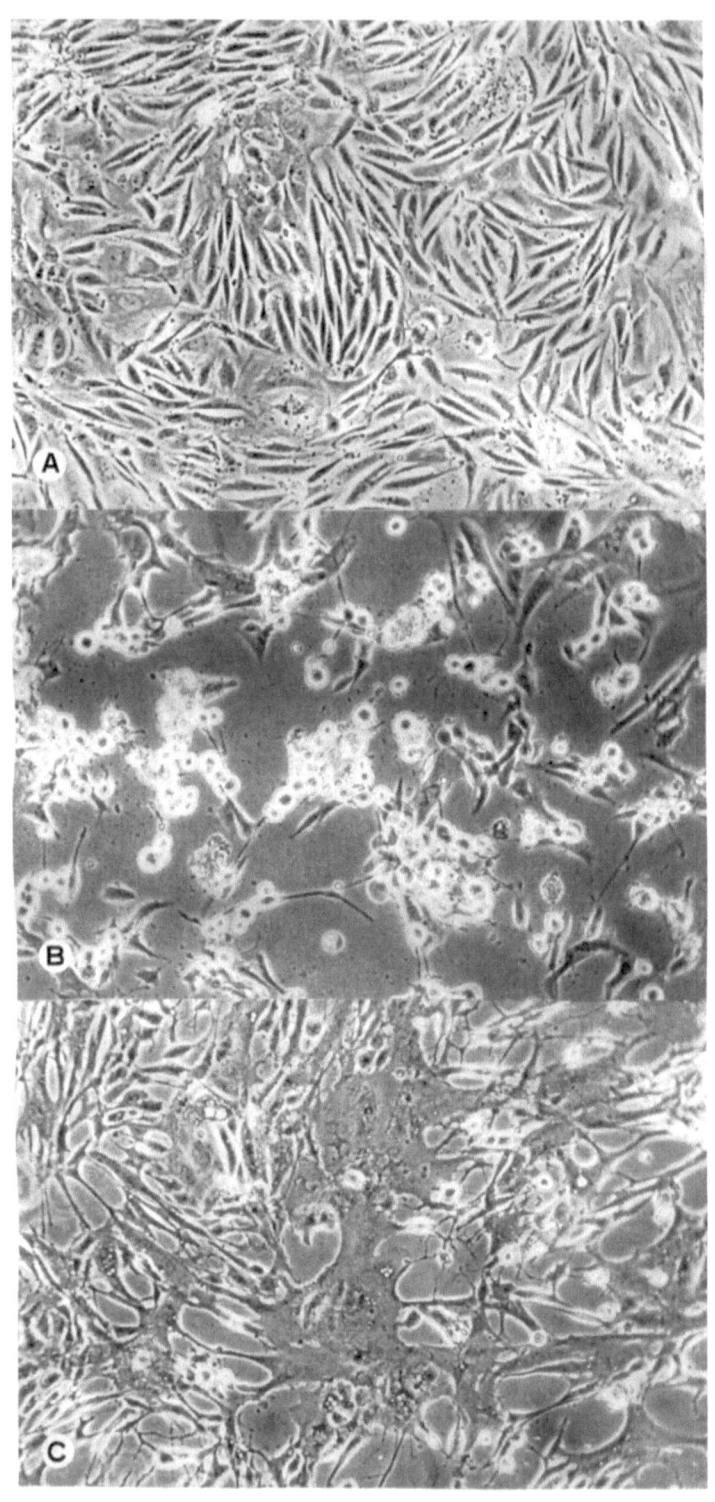

B. Intranuclear Alterations

The development of the intranuclear inclusion, as observed by staining with hematoxylin and eosin and by microcinematography, is approximately the same for herpes simplex virus and pseudorabies virus, the precise temporal relationships varying for each virus-cell system (CROUSE et al., 1950; WOLMAN and BEHAR, 1952; SCOTT et al., 1953; KERSTING et al., 1958; BARSKI and ROBINEAUX, 1959; ROSS and ORLANS, 1958; FELGENHAUER and STAMMLER, 1962; REISSIG and KAPLAN, 1962).

The first visible sign of the nuclear lesion induced by infection of cells with either virus is a change in the appearance of the nucleoli. These structures lose their optical homogeneity, become somewhat less opaque, lobulated, and finally granulated; they develop a ragged appearance and disappear by dissolution and disintegration. The normal chromatin network of the nucleus gradually becomes finely granular. Later, clear areas appear in the central zone of the nucleoplasm and as these areas increase in size, the chromatin becomes condensed in coarse strands and is displaced to the periphery of the nucleus. [The margination of the chromatin has also been demonstrated by radioautography: cellular DNA labeled with tritiated thymidine prior to infection becomes displaced gradually during the infective process and appears at the periphery of the nucleus (MUNK and SAUER, 1964)]. In the central zone of the nucleus a single homogeneous inclusion body, which results from the coalescence of small homogeneous masses, and which is Feulgen-positive, can be seen. Finally, the inclusion body shrinks and is surrounded by a halo, the typical type A inclusion of COWDRY (1934) (see Fig. 9). At this stage, the inclusion has become Feulgen-negative and eosinophilic. The halo is an artifact of fixation and is not present in living, unfixed cells (BARSKI and ROBINEAUX, 1959).

In a more detailed cytochemical analysis of HeLa cells infected with herpes simplex virus, using toluidine blue-molybdate stain, the first change LOVE and WILDY (1963) were able to detect was an enlargement of the nucleolini, the minute ribonucleoprotein granules in the nucleolus. The enlarged nucleolini were extruded into the nucleoplasm to form the so-called B-bodies. These developments occurred within 30 minutes after infection; by 3 hours, the nucleoprotein of the *pars amorpha* of the nucleolus appeared to diffuse into the adjacent nucleoplasm where the deoxynucleoproteins began to coalesce to form eventually the classical type A inclusion body. These A bodies displaced both the B-bodies and the nucleoli and, in time, filled the nucleus. Within about 6 hours after infection, minute granules containing RNA, DNA and non-histone proteins appeared inside the A bodies, increased in number during the period of virus increase, and then disappeared at the late stages of infection.

The development of the intranuclear inclusions produced in rabbit kidney cells infected with pseudorabies virus consists of two distinct stages (REISSIG and KAPLAN, 1962). During the first stage, small eosinophilic, Feulgen-negative patches appear; this process is independent of the synthesis of DNA and occurs in infected cells treated with 5-fluorouracil, as well as in untreated cells. The

Fig. 8. Cytopathic effect of herpes simplex and pseudorabies viruses on monolayers of rabbit kidney cells. A, noninfected cells; B, herpes simplex virus, rounding of the infected cells; C, pseudorabies virus, syncytia formation, ×100. Phase contrast. From A. S. KAPLAN and A. E. VATTER, Virology 7, 394 (1959).

second stage, which involves the formation of the large Feulgen-positive inclusions, develops only in cells in which the synthesis of DNA has not been inhibited, and does not appear in cells treated with 5-fluorouracil.

C. Chromosomal Alterations

Herpes simplex virus induces chromosomal aberrations following the infection of *in vitro* cultures of the aneuploid MCH line of Chinese hamster *(Cricetelus griseus)* cells (HAMPAR and ELLISON, 1961 and 1963). In the surviving cells,

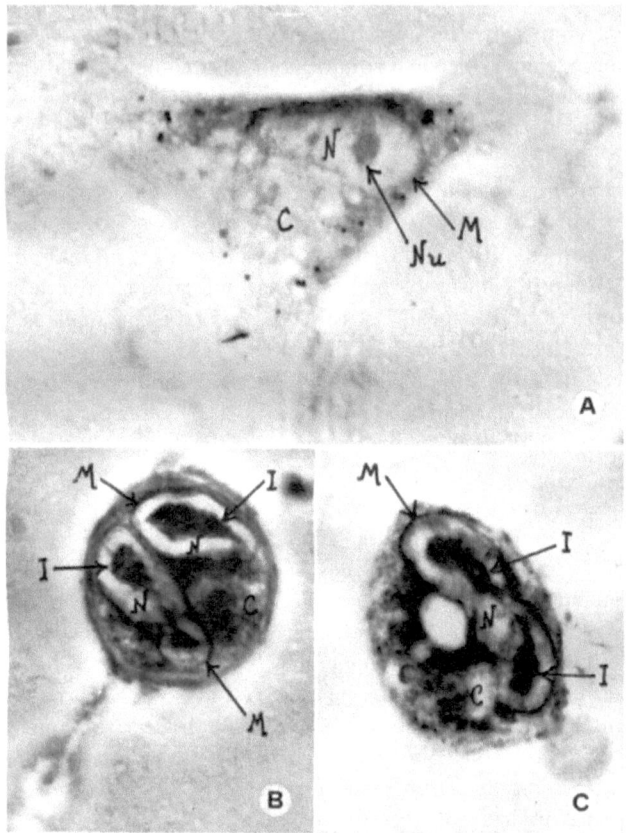

Fig. 9. Nuclear division in single rabbit kidney cells infected with pseudorabies virus. C, cytoplasm; N, nucleus; Nu, nucleolus; I, intranuclear inclusion; M, nuclear membrane.
A. A single living rabbit kidney cell photographed before virus inoculation. The cell has only one nucleus.
B. The same cell shown in A, fixed and stained with a crystal violet-citric acid solution 10 hours after infection. The cell is now binucleated and both nuclei have intranuclear inclusions.
C. Another cell, fixed and stained 10 hours after infection, which shows an elongated nucleus markedly restricted and containing an intranuclear inclusion. × 1,000. Phase contrast.
From M. REISSIG and A. S. KAPLAN, Virology 11, 1 (1960).

new breaks appear for several generations after infection, indicating that an agent causing breaks may persist in the infected cultures for some time. An increased incidence of chromosomal breaks occurs also in diploid lines of Chinese hamster cells infected with herpes simplex virus (STICH et al., 1964; RAPP and HSU, 1965).

The distribution of the breaks in the chromosomes is non-random and structural abnormalities appear in specific areas of the chromosomes. The breaks are located at loci which are similar to those caused by BUdR, hydroxylamine, and X-irradiation (HSU and SOMERS, 1961; SOMERS and HSU, 1962), suggesting that the location of the breaks is a property of the cell, not of the virus. However, chromosomal lesions will not occur in the cells of cultures inoculated with virus inactivated by heat, ultraviolet irradiation, or virus specific antibody (HAMPAR and ELLISON, 1963; TANZER et al., 1964; BOIRON et al., 1966), and it seems that these lesions occur only after the virus has replicated in the cultures (RAPP and HSU, 1965; MAZZONE and YERGANIAN, 1963). These observations suggest that the chromosomal damage to the cells is a secondary effect resulting from metabolic alterations in the culture due to virus infection and replication.

VII. Metabolism of Infected Cells

Information on the metabolism of the nucleic acids and proteins in virus-infected cells is fundamental to an understanding of the mechanisms of virus synthesis and assembly; it may also aid in the understanding of some of the causes that underlie cellular pathology and may provide a rational approach to the chemotherapy of virus infection.

Studies on host-virus interactions at the chemical level stem chiefly from the pioneer experiments of COHEN (1949), HERSHEY (1956), and others whose work has provided a wealth of information about many of the biochemical details of the infective process in bacteriophage-infected bacteria. Among other things, one of the chief reasons for the spectacular success in the biochemical analysis of infected bacteria is the fact that the methodology of phage experiments is highly quantitative. The earlier experiments on the biochemistry of animal virus infections made use of virus-infected animals and the results of these experiments are difficult to interpret. However, since the advent of cell culture techniques and the plaque assay method for the study of animal viruses, observations on the biochemical changes in animal cells which follow virus infection can now be regarded with more confidence.

A. Technical Problems in the Chemical Analysis of Cells Infected with the Herpes Viruses

An analysis of the changes in the rate of synthesis of DNA, RNA, and protein in infected cells presents several pitfalls, and care must be exercised in the choice of methods. Virus-infected cells, particularly those infected with viruses that induce the formation of syncytia, appear to be more frangible than noninfected cells and the cytoplasmic contents of cells broken as a result of manipulation will be lost to the supernatant fluids upon sedimentation of the intact cells and of the nuclei. Moreover, cell counts of syncytial masses are meaningless. Hence, a procedure which ensures total recovery must be used in order to obtain proper values for the estimation of the macromolecular composition of virus-infected cells (KAPLAN and BEN-PORAT, 1959).

The physiological state of the cell at the time of infection also influences the results one obtains when studying the changes in the rate of synthesis of nucleic acids and proteins. Cells infected in logarithmic phase have a high background of synthesis of cellular components and a high level of activity of enzymes; nondividing cells in stationary phase, on the other hand, have a low background of cellular synthesis. Infection will therefore affect the rate of overall synthesis of macromolecules in a different way in logarithmically growing and in stationary phase cells (KAPLAN and BEN-PORAT, 1960).

Colorimetric methods for the estimation of the amount of DNA per cell are relatively insensitive, and changes in the rate of synthesis of macromolecules in virus-infected cells are more readily detected by following the incorporation of radioactive isotopes. However, the amount of radioactive precursor incorporated will reflect not only the rate of macromolecular synthesis, but also will be influenced by the size of the acid-soluble intracellular pool of the precursor used. Care must therefore be taken, when evaluating the results, to be certain that the rate of incorporation of the radioisotope reflects the rate of synthesis of the macromolecule under investigation.

B. DNA Synthesis
1. Total Synthesis

The amount of DNA in HeLa cells was shown to increase after infection with herpes simplex virus. An increase in DNA per cell was noted between 6 and 9 hours after infection, before any increase in infectious virus could be observed. By 72 hours, the cells possessed nearly twice the normal content of DNA (NEWTON and STOKER, 1958; NEWTON et al., 1962).

When rabbit kidney cells in stationary phase are infected with pseudorabies virus there is also an increase in the amount of DNA per cell. However, monolayer cultures of rabbit kidney cells in logarithmic phase infected with pseudorabies virus show no change in their content of DNA, as measured by the diphenylamine reaction (KAPLAN and BEN-PORAT, 1960).

The pattern of incorporation of thymidine-2-^{14}C of infected cells displayed by monolayer cultures of rabbit kidney cells is, as expected, dependent upon the physiological state of the cells at the time of infection. Noninfected monolayer cultures of rabbit kidney cells in stationary phase incorporate little or no thymidine. As early as two hours after inoculation with pseudorabies virus, there is an increase in the amount of thymidine-2-^{14}C incorporated per hour into DNA. By about ten hours after infection, the rate of incorporation is about twenty times greater in the infected than in the noninfected cells. If thymidine-2-^{14}C is added at the time of infection and the total amount of label incorporated into the DNA of these cells at the end of the pseudorabies virus growth cycle is compared to that of noninfected cells treated identically, the infected cells will be found to incorporate ten to twenty times more labeled thymidine than the noninfected cells. The same results are obtained when the incorporation of adenine-8-^{14}C or ^{32}phosphorus into DNA is measured. One PFU is sufficient to produce a maximal increase in the rate of DNA synthesis in a rabbit kidney cell. Furthermore, every PFU is capable of inducing this response and every cell capable of giving rise to one PFU is also able to respond by an increase in the rate of synthesis of DNA. Since about 90% of the cells are able to synthesize infectious virus, it has been concluded that practically every cell present in confluent monolayers is capable of responding to infection with an increase in the rate of DNA synthesis (KAPLAN and BEN-PORAT, 1960).

The amount of thymidine-2-^{14}C incorporated into the DNA of infected and noninfected cells in logarithmic phase is approximately the same when the labeled compound is added at the time of infection and incorporation is allowed to proceed throughout the infective process (KAPLAN and BEN-PORAT, 1963). A difference in the rates of DNA synthesis between the two can be detected only

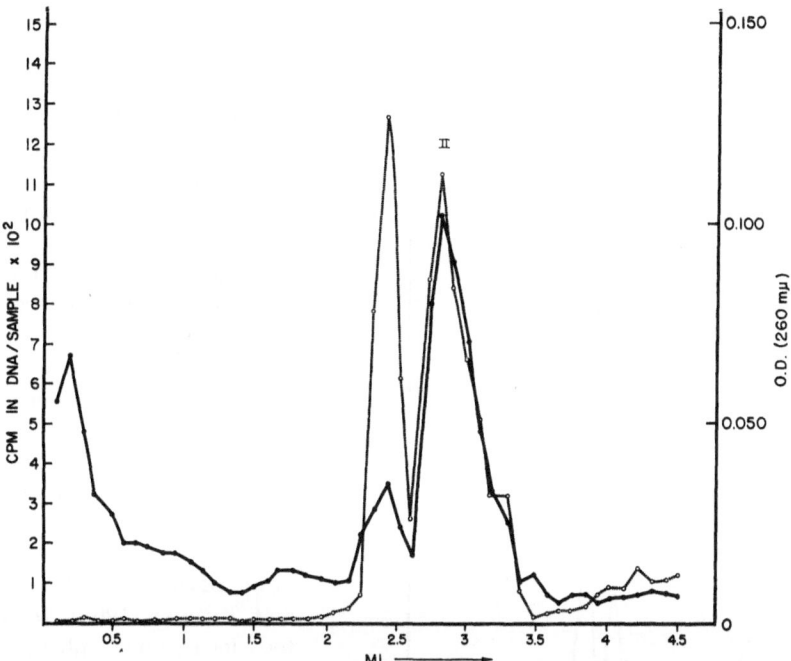

Fig. 10. Separation of cellular from viral DNA by centrifugation in a density gradient of cesium chloride. Incubation of the cells before and after infection was carried out in medium containing 2 μc of ^{32}P and 50 μg of ^{31}P per milliliter. The bottom of the centrifuge tube (highest density) is at the left, the top of the tube (lowest density) at the right. Optical density, solid line and filled circles; radioactivity, broken line and open circles. Peak I is viral DNA; peak II is cellular DNA. From A. S. KAPLAN and T. BEN-PORAT, Virology 19, 205 (1963).

by "pulse-labeling" experiments, i.e. if thymidine-2-^{14}C is added at various times during the infective process and the cells are allowed to incorporate the labeled compound for one hour prior to harvest. Using this procedure, it was found that after infection of rabbit kidney cells in logarithmic phase with pseudorabies virus there was a suppression of thymidine-2-^{14}C uptake for the first five hours; thereafter the rate of incorporation began to increase (KAPLAN and BEN-PORAT, 1960). A similar effect has been reported by NEWTON et al. (1962) for HeLa cells infected with herpes simplex virus.

2. Type of DNA Synthesized by the Infected Cells

The type of DNA (cellular or viral) synthesized by infected cells may be readily identified because these two types of DNA differ considerably in base composition, a property that permits their separation by centrifugation in a density gradient of cesium chloride, as illustrated in Fig. 10.

The relative amounts of cellular and viral DNA synthesized at different stages of the infective process in pseudorabies virus-infected cells was determined by labeling the DNA synthesized by the infected cells at various times after infection and separating viral DNA from cellular DNA by isopycnic centrifugation in cesium chloride. Each type of DNA was identified by base composition; the amount of radioactive label associated with each kind of DNA was determined. Since only the DNA synthesized during the labeling period is radioactive, the relative amounts of viral and cellular DNA synthesized during the labeling period will be proportional to the amount of label incorporated into each and can thus be ascertained. Using this technique, it was found that cells infected in stationary phase synthesized viral DNA only (BEN-PORAT and KAPLAN, 1963). In infected logarithmic phase cells there were changing rates of cellular and viral DNA synthesis at different times after infection. There was a gradual decrease after infection in the rate of incorporation of thymidine into cellular DNA as infection proceeded, and by 7 to 8 hours after inoculation, the cells infected with pseudorabies virus no longer synthesized cellular DNA. Concurrently, there was an increase in the incorporation of thymidine into viral DNA (see Fig. 11).

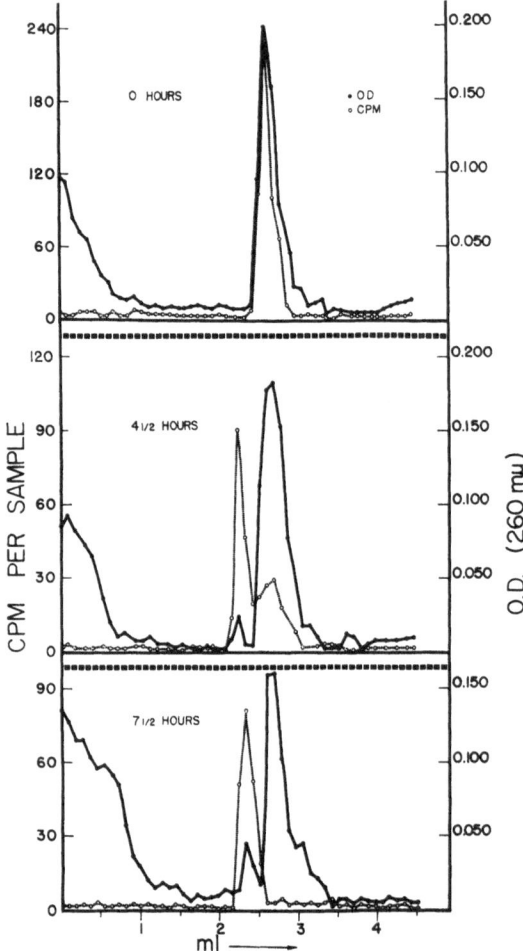

Fig. 11. The decrease in the rate of incorporation of thymidine-2-^{14}C into cellular DNA and the increase in the rate of its incorporation into viral DNA with time of infection, as determined in cesium chloride density gradients. Optical density, solid line and filled circles; radioactivity, broken line and open circles. Viral DNA is the peak on the left, cellular DNA on the right. Note that at time zero, all the radioactivity is associated with the cellular DNA, indicating that at this time only cellular DNA is being synthesized; by 7.5 hours all the radioactivity is associated with viral DNA, indicating that now only viral DNA is being synthesized. From A. S. KAPLAN and T. BEN-PORAT, Virology 19, 205 (1963).

Similar experiments have been carried out in cells infected with herpes simplex virus (ROIZMAN and ROANE, 1964; RUSSELL et al., 1964). After inoculation, a new type of DNA with a buoyant density corresponding to that of viral DNA (and therefore presumably viral DNA) made its appearance in the virus-infected cells. As is the case in pseudorabies virus-infected cells, as infection proceeded the rate of synthesis of cellular DNA decreased and there was a concomitant increase in the rate of viral DNA synthesis.

Since the DNA of all organisms studied is replicated in a semi-conservative manner, it was reasonable to assume that the DNA of animal viruses would also replicate in this fashion. This was shown to be the case for pseudorabies virus DNA by the following procedure. Rabbit kidney cells infected with pseudorabies virus were incubated in the presence of BUdR, so that the viral DNA synthesized by the cells would contain bromouracil in both strands of DNA and its buoyant density would be characteristically increased. The pattern of replication of this BU-containing DNA was then examined by removing the BUdR from the medium and incubating the infected cells in the presence of thymidine, so that the DNA formed thereafter would contain thymidine. By analysis in cesium chloride density gradients in the analytical centrifuge, it was found that hybrid viral DNA containing BU-DNA in one strand and thymidine-DNA in the other was formed in these cells, showing that the DNA of pseudorabies virus replicates semi-conservatively, *i.e.*, upon replication, the two strands of a viral DNA molecule separate and each serves as a template for the formation of a second strand. This experiment also showed that progeny viral DNA that had been synthesized by the infected cell can, in turn, replicate and indicates that, in principle, pseudorabies virus DNA replicates in a geometric fashion (KAPLAN and BEN-PORAT, 1964).

The rate of viral DNA synthesis in the rabbit kidney cells infected with pseudorabies virus increases, as shown above, with time after infection. Since pseudorabies viral DNA replicates in a geometric fashion, this increasing rate may be interpreted as being a reflection of the exponential mode of synthesis of viral DNA within the cell in which the number of DNA molecules available for replication determines the rate of DNA synthesis. However, this is not the case, as shown by the fact that the infected cells acquire the ability to synthesize viral DNA at increasing rates even when the accumulation of viral DNA molecules in these cells is inhibited (KAPLAN and BEN-PORAT, 1966b).

C. RNA Synthesis
1. Total Synthesis

Infection of cells with pseudorabies or herpes simplex viruses results in a decrease in the rate of synthesis of RNA. The incorporation of uridine-2-^{14}C or adenine-8-^{14}C into the RNA of rabbit kidney cells in logarithmic phase infected with pseudorabies virus is inhibited and by 8 hours after infection these cells incorporate about one-fifth as much uridine as noninfected cultures (KAPLAN and BEN-PORAT, 1960). A decrease in the incorporation of labeled uridine into RNA has also been observed in cells infected with herpes simplex virus (ROIZMAN et al., 1965; HAY et al., 1966; FLANAGAN, 1967).

2. Type of RNA Synthesized by Infected Cells

An analysis by means of sucrose gradients of the type of RNA synthesized by BHK21 cells infected with herpes simplex virus (HAY et al., 1966) showed that incorporation into RNA of labeled precursor was largely confined to material that had a sedimentation constant of 20S. This RNA hybridized specifically with herpes simplex virus DNA and presumably represents viral messenger RNA.

In addition to the 20S RNA, HAY et al. (1966) also found that herpes simplex virus-infected cells synthesized RNA with a sedimentation constant of 4S. SUBAK-SHARPE and his associates (1965 and 1966b) found 4S RNA present in BHK21 cells infected with herpes simplex virus that was different from the 4S RNA present in noninfected cells and formed RNase-resistant hybrids with viral DNA. However, the synthesis of host-specific 4S RNA was not arrested in these cells. This finding suggests that some of the 4S RNA synthesized by the infected cells is specified by the virus. The virus-specific molecules of 4S RNA possessed many of the attributes of transfer RNA. Chromatographic analysis on methyl-albumin-kieselgur columns suggested that a new or modified transfer RNA specific for arginine was present in the infected cells. The fact that a new transfer RNA is coded by the incoming viral genome, modifying the translation mechanism of the host cells, is an event that was predictable from the base composition of herpes simplex virus DNA which differs considerably from that of the host BHK21 cells and by the analysis of the pattern of nearest neighbor base sequences (SUBAK-SHARPE et al., 1966a).

D. Protein Synthesis
1. Total Synthesis

In contrast to the synthesis of DNA and RNA, there is little obvious change in the overall rate of protein synthesis in cells infected with pseudorabies virus or with herpes simplex virus. Rabbit kidney cells infected with pseudorabies virus do not show much change in the rate of protein synthesis as measured by colorimetric methods, or by pulse-labeling of the cells with ^{14}C-labeled leucine (KAPLAN and BEN-PORAT, 1959; HAMADA and KAPLAN, 1965). A slight decrease in the incorporation of labeled amino acids into protein has been reported for HEp-2 cells infected with herpes simplex virus (ROIZMAN et al., 1965; SYDISKIS and ROIZMAN, 1966). The effect of infection of cells with these viruses on the incorporation of amino acids into protein will probably vary to some extent, depending on the strain of virus, the host cells, the physiological state of the cells, and the labeled amino acid used.

2. Type of Proteins Synthesized by the Infected Cells

Infected cells synthesize at least two types of virus specific proteins: (1) structural proteins; i.e., proteins that become part of mature virus, and (2) non-structural proteins.

The formation of viral proteins has been studied by following the appearance in cells infected with herpes simplex virus of complement-fixing antigens that react specifically with antiserum prepared against this virus. In BHK21 or in HeLa cells a rise in the complement-fixing antigens can be detected well before the formation of infectious virus begins, and most of these antigens remain in a soluble form and do not become associated with mature viral particles (GOLD et al., 1963; RUSSELL et al., 1964).

The formation of virus-specific proteins in cells infected with pseudorabies virus has also been studied using an indirect precipitation test (HAMADA and

KAPLAN, 1965). In this method, infected cells are supplied with isotopically-labeled amino acids, so that the proteins synthesized by the cells are labeled. The viral antigens are reacted with specific γ-globulin; this complex is precipitated by antisera against the γ-globulin. The amount of radioactivity associated with the precipitate is a measure of the amount of antigen synthesized by the cell. By this method and by the use of appropriate sera, it was found that cellular protein synthesis was inhibited and by two hours after infection viral structural proteins began to be synthesized by the cells. The synthesis of these proteins preceded the formation of mature virus and continued until the end of the virus growth cycle. Immediately after their synthesis, viral structural proteins were not associated with viral particles, and could not be sedimented at centrifugal forces at which viral particles normally sediment. As the infectious cycle progressed, these proteins became associated with structures (most likely viral particles) which were sedimentable at these forces.

In both herpes simplex virus- and pseudorabies virus-infected cells antigens are formed which react with antiserum against mature virus but which do not become part of the mature viral particles. In herpes simplex virus-infected cells most of these antigens remain soluble; in pseudorabies virus-infected cells, only 35% of these antigens remain soluble. Whether these are viral structural proteins that are synthesized in excess of the amount required for the formation of viral particles, or whether the antiserum against mature virus also reacts with non-structural virus-induced proteins is not known.

The formation of nonstructural viral proteins in the infected cells was demonstrated by an indirect precipitation test using serum prepared against extracts of infected cells. During the early stages of the infective process in pseudorabies virus-infected cells, proteins which bear no precursor relationship to the viral particles (i.e., are not integrated into viral particles) are formed (HAMADA and KAPLAN, 1965). These proteins differ antigenically from the proteins found associated with viral particles and may include enzymes formed within the cell after virus infection.

Recently, the antigens of herpes simplex virus have been characterized using gel immunodiffusion and acrylamide gel immunoelectrophoresis (TOKUMARU, 1965; WATSON et al., 1966). Highly virus-specific antisera indicated the presence of at least ten to twelve different virus-specific antigens of varying size in extracts of infected cells. The relationship between these antigens and the structural proteins of the virus is, however, not yet clear.

E. Site of Synthesis of Viral Components
1. Viral DNA

Since cells in stationary phase synthesize viral DNA only (see above), it is possible to follow the site of formation of this DNA by radioautography. Studies of this type have revealed that viral DNA is synthesized within the nucleus, specifically within the intranuclear inclusion (MUNK and SAUER, 1963).

2. Viral Proteins

Virus-specific protein, as detected by staining with fluorescent antibody, was observed by LEBRUN (1956) to make its first appearance as a tiny spot in the nucleus of HEp-2 cells infected with herpes simplex virus. This was followed by the formation of more of these spherical areas and the gradual development of a network of antigenic protein within the nucleus. Eventually, the nucleus was filled with a large homogeneous region containing viral antigen. Later, viral antigen spilled over into the cytoplasm and the amount of antigenic material decreased in the nucleus.

The same sequence of events has been reported to occur in chick embryo cells infected with pseudorabies virus: viral antigen, detected with fluorescent antiserum, first appeared in the nucleus and subsequently moved to the cytoplasm (ALBRECHT et al., 1963).

A different location in the cell where viral antigen, as detected by specific fluorescent antiserum, first appears has also been reported. Thus, ROIZMAN (1961), who used the same cell-virus system as LEBRUN (1956), and NII and KAMAHORA (1963), who used the FL strain of human amniotic cells and the L strain of mouse fibroblast cells, did not observe intranuclear fluorescence; instead, they reported that viral antigen first appeared at the nuclear membrane and, as infection proceeded, moved to the cytoplasm. In point of fact, some workers have observed fluorescence simultaneously in the nucleus and in the cytoplasm (ROSS and ORLANS, 1958; MUNK and FISCHER, 1965).

These conflicting results may be due to the fact that different preparations of antiserum against infectious virus may be active against different viral components. Thus, in one case, the antisera may have reacted mainly with the viral capsid, and in the other, mainly with the outer membrane or envelope which the virus acquires as it leaves the nucleus (see below).

The fluorescent antibody technique has the limitation that by this method one locates the site of *accumulation*, but not the site of *synthesis*, of viral antigen. It is therefore not clear from these experiments whether the viral capsid proteins (which presumably accumulate in the nucleus, since the aggregation of a capsid takes place there) are indeed synthesized in the nucleus or whether, like most cellular proteins, these proteins are synthesized in the cytoplasm and thereafter migrate to the nucleus.

That some viral-specified proteins may be made on the cytoplasmic polysomes was suggested by the experiments of SYDISKIS and ROIZMAN (1966), who showed that infection of HEp-2 cells with herpes simplex virus caused the breakdown and subsequent reformation of these polysomes.

In pseudorabies virus-infected cells, it was shown that at least some structural proteins are synthesized in the cytoplasm and find their way to the nucleus (FUJIWARA and KAPLAN, 1967). Infected and noninfected cells were labeled at a time when the infected cells synthesize mostly viral proteins and the cytoplasmic fraction was separated from the nuclear fraction. Essentially no difference between infected and noninfected cells was observed in the distribution of radioactivity in the fractions which would indicate that the site of protein synthesis in infected and noninfected cells is the same. Since most of the proteins in noninfected cells are synthesized in the cytoplasm, the same must be true also for infected cells. Furthermore, a flow of labeled proteins from the cytoplasm to the nucleus could be detected in the infected cells during a pulse-chase experiment. Since these experiments were carried out when most of the proteins made by the cells were destined to become part of the viral particles, these results indicate that the viral structural proteins are probably synthesized in the cytoplasm and find their way to the nucleus of the infected cell.

F. Virus Assembly

In the bacteria-bacteriophage systems, it has been established that the synthesis of bacteriophage DNA precedes the formation of intact virus and that there is within the infected cell a pool of vegetative (replicating and recombining) DNA from which DNA is withdrawn at random to be enclosed within the viral particles. Thus, the formation of all the components of the viral particles is not simultaneous but the components are made separately and the virus is assembled later. Information about the mode of synthesis of the herpes viruses is less complete. However, all the available information points to a mechanism of synthesis similar to that of bacteriophage.

1. Kinetics of Synthesis and Assembly of Viral Components

As mentioned above, because of differences in base composition, it is relatively simple to follow the time course of viral DNA formation in cells infected with either pseudorabies virus or herpes simplex virus. In pseudorabies virus-infected cells, viral DNA is first detected about 2 hours after infection and is synthesized at increasing rates up until about 9 to 10 hours after infection (KAPLAN et al., 1965; KAPLAN and BEN-PORAT, 1966b). The synthesis of herpes simplex viral DNA in BHK 21 cells is first detectable about 5 hours after infection. The rate of viral DNA synthesis increases until about 7 hours and then remains constant (RUSSELL et al., 1964).

The question whether viral DNA synthesized by the infected cells at one time during the infective process becomes part of mature virus assembled later in the infectious cycle was answered by the following experiment. The viral DNA made by infected stationary phase cells between three and four hours after infection was labeled, and it was shown that as the number of infectious viral particles produced by the cells increased, the amount of radioactive DNA associated with the virus also increased. Thus, DNA synthesized by the infected cells early in the infectious cycle was used for the formation of viral particles assembled later in the cycle. However, only about 15% of the DNA made between 3 and 4 hours after infection became associated with mature viral particles and this finding raised the question whether DNA synthesized early during the infection (when few viral particles are formed) has a smaller chance to be integrated into viral particles than DNA synthesized later in the cycle. It was found that this is not the case and that DNA made at various stages of the infectious cycle has an equal chance to contribute to the formation of viral particles maturing at any later time in the virus growth cycle. Thus, there is in the infected cells a pool from which precursor DNA is withdrawn at random for the formation of viral particles. Viral DNA is made in excess and only about 12% of the total viral DNA synthesized by the cells becomes associated with the viral particles (BEN-PORAT and KAPLAN, 1963).

Viral protein synthesis in both herpes simplex virus- and pseudorabies virus-infected cells precedes the formation of infectious virus and viral proteins seem

4*

to be made in excess of the amount required for the formation of mature virus (RUSSELL et al., 1964; HAMADA and KAPLAN, 1965). Furthermore, immediately after their synthesis, viral proteins are not associated with viral particles and assembly takes place at the later stages of the infective process (HAMADA and KAPLAN, 1965).

2. Site of Virus Assembly

The development of intranuclear inclusions in cells infected with pseudorabies virus or herpes simplex virus would seem to point to the nucleus as the site of virus assembly. A relatively large body of evidence has accumulated indicating that this assumption is correct.

Thus, GRAY and SCOTT (1954) isolated nuclei from the liver cells of chick embryos infected with herpes simplex virus and found virus associated with the nuclei. Although the method they employed left the nuclear fraction contaminated with cytoplasmic material, the experiments on the cellular distribution of infectious virus at various times after infection showed that the amount of infectious virus in the nucleus decreased as the infective process proceeded and eventually practically all of the virus left the nucleus. It is pertinent to note here that the intranuclear inclusions are Feulgen-positive early in the infectious cycle indicating the presence of DNA, presumably viral DNA, whereas the fully developed inclusions at the end of the growth cycle are Feulgen-negative and do not contain virus (SCOTT et al., 1953; CROUSE et al., 1950; WOLMAN and BEHAR, 1952).

The most direct evidence that herpes simplex virus and pseudorabies virus are assembled within the nuclei of infected cells comes from observations made with the electron microscope. It is clear from these observations that the viral capsids are assembled in the nucleus and that after being assembled, they pass to the cytoplasm and acquire their envelopes.

At various times after infection, MORGAN et al. (1954) examined with the electron microscope thin-sections of herpes simplex virus-infected cells. These studies revealed the following sequence of events leading to the formation of herpes simplex virus. The first obvious alteration in the nuclei of the infected cells is margination of the chromatin. In or near this material dense central bodies approximately 30 to 40 mμ in diameter are formed. The central body appears to increase in diameter (40 to 50 mμ), to become somewhat less dense, and to become surrounded by a membrane 6 to 8 mμ in diameter, the entire structure being about 70 to 100 mμ in diameter. Thus, the particles observed within the nucleus have this diameter and contain one membrane. [Certain strains of herpes simplex virus can form intranuclear crystals (MORGAN et al., 1958; EPSTEIN, 1962a).] The viral particles appearing in the cytoplasm, however, possess a double membrane with a diameter of 120 to 130 mμ. From these observations, MORGAN et al. (1954) concluded that the site of viral development is in the nucleus where the initial bodies are formed and are enclosed by a single membrane; the second membrane appears to be acquired as the viral particles are released into the cytoplasm (see Fig. 1).

Later, REISSIG and MELNICK (1955) found, however, that characteristic particles of herpes-B virus, a virus related to both herpes simplex and pseudorabies viruses, possessing a double membrane could be observed within the nuclei of the infected cells. This was also found by STOKER et al. (1958) and by MORGAN et al. (1959) for herpes simplex virus. Because of the limitations inherent in the techniques these investigators employed, it was not certain whether these double membrane particles were really within the nucleus proper or within cytoplasmic invaginations of the nucleus which becomes dramatically distorted by infection. More recent studies indicate rather clearly that the viral particles present in the nucleus contain a single membrane and that they acquire a second membrane as they leave the nucleus (FALKE et al., 1959; C. MORGAN, personal communication, 1967). It appears that the viral particles will acquire their second coat from the nuclear membrane or from other membranes within the cell, as well as from the cell membrane where they can be seen budding from the cell, sometimes as particles with a triple membrane (EPSTEIN, 1962).

A detailed electron microscopic analysis by FELLUGA (1963) revealed that the course of morphological development of pseudorabies virus in pig kidney cells follows that described for herpes simplex virus.

G. Enzymology of the Virus-infected Cells
1. Levels of Enzyme Activity

Since, under certain conditions, the herpes viruses induce in infected cells an increase in the synthesis of DNA, it is not surprising to find that the infective process is accompanied by an increase in the activity of some of the enzymes required for the formation of DNA. Thus, KEIR and GOLD (1963) found that after infection of BHK 21 cells with herpes simplex virus there is an initial decline in the activity of DNA polymerase followed by an increase in activity of the enzyme of about sevenfold by 7 hours after infection; later (8 to 16 hours after infection) the activity is drastically reduced. Most of the enzyme activity is found associated with the nuclei of the infected cells. In rabbit kidney cells infected with pseudorabies virus there is also an increase in the activity of DNA polymerase, which starts between 1.5 and 2 hours after infection and continues up to about 10 hours after infection (NOHARA and KAPLAN, 1963; KAMIYA et al., 1964; KAPLAN et al., 1965). In both systems the increase in activity of DNA polymerase precedes the formation of infectious virus.

Infection with herpes simplex virus and pseudorabies virus results also in an increase in the activity of thymidine kinase and TMP kinase (NOHARA and KAPLAN, 1963; KIT and DUBBS, 1963a; HAMADA et al., 1966; KAPLAN et al., 1967). In mouse fibroblast cells (Earle's L cells) infected with herpes simplex virus, thymidine kinase activity starts to increase about 2 hours after infection and increases rapidly over the next 6 hours. The increase in the activity of thymidine kinase and of TMP kinase in rabbit kidney cells infected with pseudorabies virus parallels that of DNA polymerase, i.e., the increase is detectable about 1 to 2 hours after infection and reaches a maximum 6 hours after infection (KAMIYA et al., 1965).

The level of activity of the other kinases involved in DNA synthesis remains the same in the infected cells and in the noninfected cells (HAMADA et al., 1966). Other enzymes on the pathway of DNA synthesis which do not increase in activity after infection of cells with herpes simplex virus are thymidylate synthetase (FREARSON et al., 1965) and dihydrofolate reductase (FREARSON et al., 1966).

The effect of virus infection on the carbohydrate metabolism of the infected cells has also been examined. Thus, for example, when glucose is used as the principal substrate, HeLa cells infected with herpes simplex virus produce more organic acids, such as lactate, succinate, and pyruvate than noninfected cells. The pathways for the formation of these acids are, however, the same in infected and noninfected cells (FISHER and FISHER, 1959; FISHER and FISHER, 1961). In spite of the increase in production of organic acids after infection, there is little or no increase in hexokinase and glucose-6-phosphate dehydrogenase activity until late in infection. The increase at that time may, however, be the reflection only of changes in the permeability of the cell membranes due to virus infection and the consequent greater accumulation of substrate within the infected cells (SCOTT et al., 1961).

Infection with the herpes viruses results in drastic alterations of the normal organization of the cells, as described above, ending in cell necrosis and dissolution. These visually observable effects, it was thought, might result from the activity of the hydrolytic enzymes contained within the lysosomes, the particles that are enclosed within a membrane and located in the cytoplasm (DE DUVE, 1963; NOVIKOFF, 1963). Yet, when KB cells are infected with herpes simplex virus, there is only a minimal increase in the activity of the lysosomal enzymes, β-glucuronidase, "acid" DNase, and acid phosphatase (FLANAGAN, 1966). On the other hand, there is a marked increase in the activity of two "alkaline" DNases in HeLa cells infected with herpes simplex virus; one of these enzymes hydrolyzes native DNA optimally at pH 9.2 and the other, denatured DNA optimally at pH 9.5 (McAUSLAN et al., 1965).

2. Mechanism of Increase in Enzyme Activity

The increase in the activity of some of the enzymes after infection, as described above, may be due to the synthesis in the infected cells of new proteins. Whether or not these proteins are different from the proteins performing the same functions in noninfected cells is of considerable importance and has been the subject of many studies. This information may aid in the understanding of the respective roles played by the viral genome and the host cell genome in the control of this part of the infective process. In attempts to answer this question, the physicochemical and antigenic character of the DNA polymerases and thymidine kinases present in infected and noninfected cells have been analyzed.

Evidence has been obtained that three enzymes involved in DNA synthesis, the activities of which are increased by infection, possess different physicochemical characteristics from the enzymes performing the same function in noninfected cells.

DNA polymerase present in BHK 21 cells or in HEp-2 cells infected with herpes simplex virus appears to be more thermostable than the enzymes from noninfected cells. Furthermore, the enzymes from infected and noninfected cells display different magnesium ion requirements for their in vitro reaction, as well as different primer requirements (KEIR et al., 1966a). The enzyme present in the infected cells also differs in its antigenic properties from the DNA polymerase present in noninfected cells (KEIR et al., 1966b). The DNA polymerases present in pseudorabies virus-infected and noninfected cells, on the other hand, cross-reacted with the heterologous serum and could not be differentiated by this method, indicating that the enzymes from the two sources have some antigenic structures in common. The differences in the results obtained with herpes simplex virus and pseudorabies virus may be due to differences in the method of preparation of the specific antisera.

The thymidine kinase that appears in cells infected with pseudorabies virus and herpes simplex virus has also been subjected to the same kind of analysis as DNA polymerase. Thus, HAMADA et al. (1966) showed that the thymidine kinase produced in rabbit kidney cells infected with pseudorabies virus is immunologically distinct from the enzyme present in noninfected cells. This was also found to be the case for the enzyme present in BHK 21 cells infected with herpes simplex virus (KLEMPERER et al., 1967). The thymidine kinase present in the herpes simplex virus-infected cells also differs from the enzyme present in noninfected cells in other characteristics: it has a low pH optimum, is relatively insensitive to inhibition by thymidine triphosphate, and is more thermostable than the host cell enzyme. The thymidine kinase present in the virus-infected cells also differs from the enzyme present in noninfected cells in its Km value and inhibition by trifluoromethyl-2'-deoxyuridine (KIT et al., 1967).

The TMP kinases present in pseudorabies virus-infected and noninfected rabbit kidney cells differ in two of their characteristics: the enzyme from infected cells is more thermostable than the enzyme from noninfected cells, and, in contrast to the latter, does not require substrate for stabilization (NOHARA and KAPLAN, 1963). The stability in the absence of added substrate of TMP kinase from infected cells is not due to a larger pool of thymidine derivatives in these cells, because the enzyme remains stable even after dialysis (KAPLAN et al., 1967).

All this evidence would seem to indicate that DNA polymerase, thymidine kinase, and TMP kinase present in virus-infected cells are new and different proteins and are possibly coded by the viral genome. However, the fact that enzymes from infected and noninfected cells differ in many of their physicochemical properties does not constitute compelling proof for their *de novo* synthesis in the virus-infected cells. Instead, the increase in the activity of the enzymes may be the result of the creation in the infected cells of conditions in which the enzymes present in the cell at the time of infection are stabilized by substrate (BOJARSKI and HIATT, 1960; WRIGHT, 1960; WEISSMAN et al., 1960; LITTLE-FIELD, 1965) or released from inhibitory control mechanisms (GERHARDT and PARDEE, 1963; CHANGEUX, 1963; FREUNDLICH and UMBARGER, 1963). For example, it is known that thymidine kinase isolated from the same source will have different Km and Ki values depending upon the state of aggregation of the enzyme (BRESNICK et al., 1966). Even the different antigenicity displayed by the DNA polymerase and thymidine kinase from infected cells, which appears to indicate that infection does indeed induce the *de novo* synthesis within the cell of new and different enzyme proteins, is not a completely reliable criterion. Thus, an alteration in the antigenicity of a protein can also occur as a result of a change in its physical state: under certain conditions, the molecular form of crystalline glutamic dehydrogenase is changed from a polymer to a monomer, thereby also changing the antigenicity of the enzyme (TALAL et al., 1965). The increased activity of the enzymes in the infected cells, as well as the difference in their physico-chemical characteristics could be due, therefore, to the fact that the infective process creates conditions within the infected cells that favor a change in the physical state of the enzyme present at the time of infection, thereby changing its stability and antigenicity, and does not reflect the *de novo* synthesis of enzymes different from the ones present in noninfected cells.

As demonstrated for TMP kinase in pseudorabies virus-infected cells (KAPLAN et al., 1967), an increase in the level of activity in virus-infected cells of an enzyme with physico-chemical characteristics different from those of the same enzyme in noninfected cells does not necessarily imply that the enzyme is a new and different protein synthesized *de novo*. The increase in the level of activity of thymidylate kinase, although prevented by inhibitors of protein synthesis, is not due to the synthesis of new enzyme protein; instead the enzyme present in noninfected cells, which is normally unstable *in vitro*, seems as a result of infection to acquire new properties that confer upon it stability *in vitro*. Thus, the fact that the increase in the level of activity of DNA polymerase and thymidine kinase is prevented by the addition to the infected cells of inhibitors of protein synthesis does not necessarily indicate that the increase in activity of these enzymes is due to the formation of new enzyme protein. Protein synthesis may be required for the creation of the conditions that favor stabilization and change the physico-chemical characteristics of the enzymes present in the cells at the time of infection.

There is, however, one line of evidence demonstrating that thymidine kinase, at least, may be a new enzyme coded by the viral genome (KIT and DUBBS, 1963 a and b; DUBBS and KIT, 1964 and 1965; KIT and DUBBS, 1965). KIT and his associates have isolated a mutant of mouse fibroblast cells (strain LMTK⁻) that lacks (or has very low levels of) thymidine kinase. Infection of these mutant cells with herpes simplex virus leads to a considerable increase of thymidine kinase activity. Mutants of herpes simplex virus have been isolated that induce in the LMTK⁻ cells either very low levels of thymidine kinase or none at all. Although the thymidine kinase-less mutants of both the cells and the virus are "leaky", the results cited above provide reasonable support for the view that the thymidine kinase induced in cells by infection is a new protein coded by the virus.

One of the more interesting questions that has arisen from the studies on the enzymology of virus-infected cells is the following: what particular value to virus survival does the large increase in thymidine kinase confer to cells infected with herpes simplex virus and pseudorabies virus? The role of thymidine kinase in DNA synthesis in general has been a subject of much speculation. The function of thymidine kinase may be explained in terms of competition between anabolic and catabolic enzymatic pathways, as suggested by POTTER (1958 and 1960) and CANELLAKIS et al. (1959). An increase in the level of activity of this enzyme provides an alternate pathway for the synthesis of thymidine monophosphate. However, the results of DUBBS and KIT (1964) appear to indicate that the presence of thymidine kinase in a virus-infected cell has no survival value for the virus, because virus mutants lacking the ability to induce the formation of this enzyme grow as well as wild-type virus.

It has been established with a variety of tissues that actively growing cells contain lower levels of phosphatase than do non-growing cells (MALEY and MALEY, 1961; BELTZ, 1962; FIALA et al., 1962; EKER, 1965), and although thymidine kinase may have no survival value if infection occurs in growing cells, it may be of importance if viral DNA synthesis is to occur in resting cells. To overcome the effect of the catabolic enzymes present in the stationary phase cells, the infecting virus must establish a mechanism to ensure the accumulation of the deoxyribonucleotide triphosphates necessary for the synthesis of DNA. Thymidine kinase induced by infection with pseudorabies virus may be indeed essential if DNA synthesis is to occur in cells having a high level of phosphatase activity (KAPLAN et al., 1967). This function of thymidine kinase has also been suggested as one reason for the increased activity of this enzyme in polyoma virus-infected cells (KIT et al., 1966).

H. Control of the Infective Process

The infective process follows a well-ordered sequence of events in virus-infected cells: Virus attaches to the cells, penetrates, and after the virus has been uncoated, information from the viral genome is transcribed to messenger RNA so that all the proteins necessary to the infective process are formed; finally, viral DNA and proteins accumulate in the cell and the viral components are assembled into infectious virus which is then released from the cells. Certain processes of infection become operative and others inoperative at critical junctures of the virus growth cycle, and the basis for the molecular control of all these events is under intensive investigation at the present time.

1. Cut-off of Synthesis of Cell-specific Components

One of the first consequences of infection of cells with the viruses is the inhibition of the synthesis of cellular protein (HAMADA and KAPLAN, 1965; SYDISKIS and ROIZMAN, 1966), as well as the inhibition of the synthesis of cellular DNA (KAPLAN and BEN-PORAT, 1963; ROIZMAN and ROANE, 1964). The inhibition of the synthesis of cellular DNA is due neither to its breakdown nor to interference by the virus with the initiation of the synthesis of cellular DNA by preventing the cells from entering into the S phase (DNA synthesizing phase) of their growth cycle. This inhibition is also not due to a successful competition of viral DNA with cellular DNA to act as a template for DNA replication, nor to a greater affinity of the DNA polymerase present in virus-infected cells for viral DNA than for cellular DNA. It appears that a specific protein is responsible for the inhibition of the synthesis of cellular DNA in the infected cells. The evidence available at present indicates that this protein does not act catalytically (BEN-PORAT and KAPLAN, 1965).

The inhibition of cellular protein synthesis is probably related to the disruption of the polysomes present in the cells at the time of infection. SYDISKIS and ROIZMAN (1966) have shown that when cells are infected with herpes simplex virus, polysomes normally present in the cells are destroyed. Later, polysomes with a sedimentation constant different from the ones present in noninfected cells make their appearance. The mechanism by which polysomes are destroyed upon infection of the cells remains to be elucidated.

2. Regulation of Enzyme Activity

As described above, an increase in the activity of the enzymes thymidine kinase, thymidine monophosphate kinase and DNA polymerase occurs in cells infected with either herpes simplex virus or pseudorabies virus. The activity of these enzymes starts increasing early in the infectious cycle, reaches a maximum, and remains unchanged thereafter until the end of the infective process. This sequence of events is analogous to that observed in bacteriophage-infected bacteria. In the case of bacteriophage, the synthesis of the so-called "early" enzymes has been shown to occur in a variety of systems for a limited period of time only, unless there is interference with a mechanism which normally regulates the level of the enzymes. This interference can be achieved by ultra-violet irradiation of the infecting virus (DIRKSEN et al., 1960; DELIHAS, 1961) or when the bacteria are infected with certain amber mutants of T4 phage which do not allow the synthesis of viral DNA to proceed at a normal rate (WIBERG et al., 1962). Thus, the control of the synthesis of the early enzymes seems to be correlated with the level of progeny viral DNA.

A lack of regulation of enzyme activity can also be obtained in cells infected with the herpes viruses, if cells infected with these viruses are incubated with BUdR or IUdR, so that most of the thymidine present in the viral DNA is replaced by the halogenated compounds. Under these conditions, the increase in activity of the "early" enzymes occurs, but the normal cut-off of enzyme activity becomes inoperative (KAPLAN et al., 1965; KAMIYA et al., 1964 and 1965). The interference in the regulation of enzyme activity is probably due to the presence of IUdR or BUdR in progeny viral DNA and it seems, therefore, that the cut-off of enzyme activity is controlled by this DNA. Since in the infected cells incubated with either BUdR or IUdR, progeny viral DNA does accumulate and there is, nevertheless, interference with the regulation of the level of enzyme activity, it seems that regulation is not dependent upon the level of progeny viral DNA *per se*, but upon the presence of competent progeny viral DNA.

I. Molecular Viral Chemotherapy

The keratitis caused by herpes simplex virus is probably the first disease induced by a virus to be cured specifically by a drug (KAUFMAN et al., 1962). The chemotherapeutic agents which are effective in controlling this disease are the halogenated derivatives of thymidine, an essential component of DNA. In view of the importance of this subject, it is worth examining the configuration of thymidine and its halogenated derivatives which are used in chemotherapy, as well as the molecular basis for their chemotherapeutic action. The clinical application of these drugs to the diseases caused by herpes simplex virus and pseudorabies virus will be discussed later.

Fig. 12 shows the structural relationships between the naturally occurring compounds (deoxyuridine and thymidine or 5-methyl-deoxyuridine) and their halogenated derivatives. Substitution of a halogen for the methyl group in the 5-position has a profound effect on the chemical and biological properties of thymidine by changing its stereochemical configuration; the type and magnitude of the effect depends on the particular halogen substituted. BUdR, IUdR and, to a lesser degree, CUdR are readily incorporated in place of thymidine in DNA;

the incorporation appears to be possible because of the similarity of the dimensions of the atomic radii of iodine, bromine and chlorine to that of the CH_3 group of thymidine. Recently, a new fluorine compound, 5-trifluoromethyl-2'-deoxyuridine has been reported to be incorporated into DNA (KAUFMAN and HEIDELBERGER, 1964). FUdR, on the other hand, is not incorporated into DNA, because the size of the atomic radius of fluorine is more like that of hydrogen than that of the methyl group and it will therefore behave like an analogue of deoxyuridine rather than of thymidine. Whereas the inhibition of cell multiplication by BUdR, IUdR and CUdR is probably due, in large measure, to the incorporation of these compounds into DNA and to the consequent formation of "faulty" DNA molecules, the inhibition of DNA synthesis by FUdR results from its inhibition of the enzyme thymidylate synthetase which acts to convert deoxyuridine to thymidine (BOSCH et al., 1958; COHEN et al., 1958).

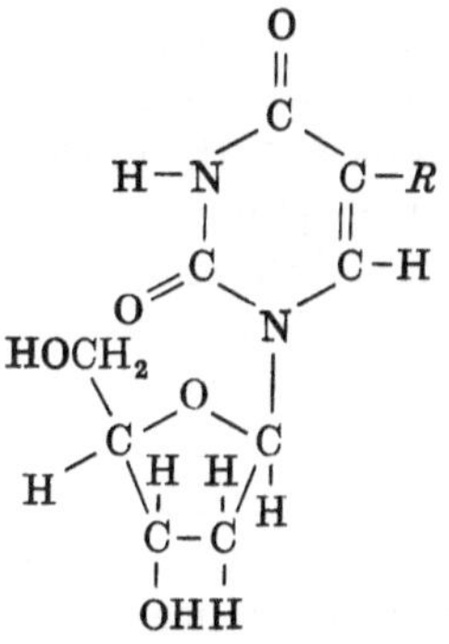

	R	Van der Waals' radius (A°)	Compound	
	H	1.20	2'-Deoxyuridine	UdR
	F	1.35	5-Fluoro-2'-deoxyuridine	FUdR
	Cl	1.80	5-Chloro-2'-deoxyuridine	CUdR
	Br	1.95	5-Bromo-2'-deoxyuridine	BUdR
	CH_3	2.00	5-Methyl-2'-deoxyuridine (Thymidine)	TdR
	I	2.15	5-Iodo-2'-deoxyuridine	IUdR
	CF_3	2.44	5-Trifluoromethyl-2'-deoxyuridine	CF_3-UdR

Fig. 12. The structural relationships of thymidine and the halogen-substituted deoxyuridines.

The nature of the inhibition of the growth of the herpes viruses by BUdR and IUdR has been studied intensively in recent years. IUdR, as well as BUdR, is incorporated into the DNA of pseudorabies virus (KAPLAN et al., 1965; KAPLAN and BEN-PORAT, 1964); viral DNA, as well as viral antigens, accumulate in the infected cells treated with these drugs. However, whereas viral particles containing BUdR-DNA are assembled in BUdR-treated cells, viral particles are not assembled in IUdR-treated cells (SMITH and DUKES, 1964; KAPLAN et al., 1965; KAPLAN and BEN-PORAT, 1966a). The lack of formation of viral particles containing IUdR-DNA is not due to a physical distortion of the DNA molecule resulting from the presence of the iodine atom *per se* in viral DNA, thereby preventing the enclosure of this DNA into viral coat proteins; instead, viral DNA containing IUdR causes the synthesis of nonfunctional proteins that are normally involved in viral assembly. IUdR-containing DNA can, however, initiate the infective process and upon replication give rise to normal, thymidine-containing DNA. Thus, the viricidal action of IUdR may be explained by the fact that it is incorporated into viral DNA and its presence in the DNA interferes with mechanisms that are essential to the normal course of events taking place during the infective process (KAPLAN and BEN-PORAT, 1966a).

Whether or not IUdR is a selective antiviral drug is an important question. Since survival of the virus is dependent upon the orderly process of virus assembly, and since IUdR prevents this process, virus replication may be especially sensitive to the replacement in viral DNA of thymidine by IUdR. However, some cellular function essential for cell division may be equally sensitive to this interchange of nucleosides in cellular DNA.

There have been contradictory reports on the relative sensitivity of virus and host cell multiplication to the drug (HANNA and WILKINSON, 1965; SMITH, 1963; EY et al., 1964; KAUFMAN, 1965). A comparison of the effect of different concentrations of IUdR on the multiplication of virus and of cells is relatively difficult, because the cycle of viral multiplication is short compared to the generation time of cells and a large number of virions is produced during each cycle. The two parameters cannot therefore be tested under identical conditions. Furthermore, if the virus is allowed to undergo several cycles of growth, mutants resistant to IUdR may appear in the drug-treated cultures.

A possible physiological basis for the antiviral specificity of IUdR may rest in the fact that infection of cells with the herpes viruses results in an increase in the level of activity of thymidine kinase. The thymidine kinase in the infected cells may have a greater affinity for IUdR than the enzyme present in non-infected cells and thereby elevate the level of phosphorylated IUdR which could then compete for incorporation into DNA with the thymidine derivatives synthesized by the cell. This possibility has been considered and has been found not to be the case (PRUSOFF et al., 1965). However, even though differences in the affinity of the thymidine kinases of infected and noninfected cells for IUdR have not been observed, the differences between the level of activities of these enzymes in the infected and noninfected cells may result in differences in the size of the pool of phosphorylated IUdR and a greater substitution of IUdR for thymidine in the DNA of infected cells than of noninfected cells would result. Considerable differences between the degree of substitution in the DNA of infected and noninfected cells have indeed been found when the cells are supplied with low concentrations of IUdR (up to about 1 µg/ml). However, the selective antiviral effect disappears when higher concentrations of the drug are used (KAPLAN and BEN-PORAT, 1967a and b). Thus, under the proper conditions, IUdR will act as a specific antiviral agent.

Another compound, Ara-C, has been reported to be as effective as IUdR in the control of herpes keratitis. This analogue of deoxycytidine is, however, slow compared to IUdR in clearing the initial infection of herpes keratitis (UNDERWOOD, 1962; KAUFMAN, 1965) and is considerably more toxic than IUdR to the host cells (KAUFMAN et al., 1964). In contrast to IUdR, Ara-C cannot be considered a selective antiviral substance, because it is more effective in inhibiting the synthesis of DNA in noninfected rabbit kidney cells than in pseudorabies virus-infected cells. The greater ability of the virus-infected cells to synthesize DNA in the presence of Ara-C is due to the fact that the drug is less efficiently phosphorylated by these cells than by noninfected cells. The low level of phosphorylation of Ara-C in the infected cells may be related to the increased activity of cytidine diphosphate reductase, the consequent accumulation of dCTP in the pool, and the feedback inhibition of deoxycytidine kinase (KAPLAN and BEN-PORAT, 1967b).

VIII. Abortive Infection

Infection of cells does not always result in the formation of infectious virus. If virus adsorbs to the cell, penetrates, and although one or more viral components are synthesized, no infectious virus is produced, this type of infection may be considered abortive. (This definition excludes nonsusceptible cells which do not adsorb virus.) An example of this kind of infection is provided by the interaction of the MP strain of herpes simplex virus with canine kidney cells (AURELIAN and ROIZMAN, 1964). Infection of the canine kidney cells with herpes simplex virus results in the production of viral antigen, interferon, and DNA which appears to be viral, and although most of the canine kidney cells do not survive infection, neither infectious virus nor viral particles are produced. Since the canine kidney cells will support the replication of pseudorabies virus, some element must be missing from these infected cells that is specific for the synthesis of herpes simplex virus. In fact, experiments indicate that in dog kidney cells, one or more structural constituents of the virus are either not made or else are nonfunctional (ROIZMAN and AURELIAN, 1965). However, the actual reasons for the abortive infection of herpes simplex virus in the canine kidney cells are not known at the present time.

IX. Pathogenesis

A. Susceptible Animals

The natural host for herpes simplex virus is man, in whom the disease caused by this virus is generally mild, although it can cause certain severe infections that will be described later. However, introduction of herpes simplex virus into susceptible animals results in severe infection. Herpes simplex virus can be transmitted experimentally to rabbits, guinea pigs, mice, rats, hamsters (WENNER, 1944), cotton rats (FLORMAN and TRADER, 1947), chick embryos (BEVERIDGE and BURNET, 1946), 1 day old chicks, and pigeons, geese and hedgehogs (REMLINGER and BAILLY, 1927; NICOLAU, 1948; VAN ROOYEN and RHODES, 1948; TOKUMARU and SCOTT, 1964).

Pseudorabies virus produces generally a mild disease in swine, its natural host, but a fatal disease in cattle. Other animals found infected in nature are dogs, cats, sheep and rats. Experimentally, pseudorabies virus can be transmitted by the inoculation of the virus to the following animals: chickens, rabbits, guinea pigs, cats, embryonated eggs, pigeons and sheep (BAILLY, 1938; GALLOWAY, 1938; GLOVER, 1939; BURNET et al., 1939; TONEVA, 1958; and TOKUMARU and SCOTT, 1964). Wild animals such as foxes, skunks, cottontail rabbits, muskrats, raccoons, badgers, woodchucks, oppossums, and deer are also susceptible to infection with pseudorabies virus (TRAINER and KARSTAD, 1963).

B. Influence of the Age of Animals on Pathogenicity of Herpes Simplex and Pseudorabies Viruses

The age of an animal at the time of infection with viruses plays an important role in the outcome of disease (BURNET, 1960; SIGEL, 1952). ANDERVONT (1929a) found that adult mice are more resistant than younger animals to infection with herpes simplex virus inoculated by routes other than intracerebral. This observation was confirmed and extended by LENNETTE and KOPROWSKI (1944): Mice 3 to 8 days of age were susceptible to extraneural inoculation of herpes simplex virus, but larger amounts of virus were required than when the virus was inoculated intracerebrally. Between 8 and 14 days of age, the mice developed resistance and some of them survived after being inoculated peripherally with large amounts of virus. After reaching 28 days of age or more, the mice appeared to be completely resistant to extraneural inoculation of herpes simplex virus.

Newborn swiss mice (1-day old) are extremely sensitive to peripheral inoculation of herpes simplex virus. In fact, these animals are more sensitive than chick embryos or rabbits to herpes simplex virus freshly isolated from human sources (KILBOURNE and HORSFALL, 1951). Newborn mice have proved to be a useful tool for the study of the pathogenesis of herpes simplex virus.

Although the difference in susceptibility to pseudorabies virus is slight between adult and young (12-day old) mice, after intracerebral, intranasal, or subcutaneous inoculation (KING, 1940), pigs, the natural host for this virus, show a decided difference in susceptibility that is age-dependent (AKKERMANS, 1963). The disease is severe in piglets up to about ten days after birth; beyond that time there is a progressive decrease in the severity of the disease. Chick embryos also succumb with encephalitis after inoculation of pseudorabies virus on the chorioallantoic membrane and so do 2 days old chicks after being inoculated subcutaneously (BANG, 1942). Adult chickens are, however, resistant to subcutaneous inoculation of the virus (SHOPE, 1931).

Thus, a clear-cut relationship exists between the age of a host and its susceptibility to the herpes viruses. However, the reason for this age-dependent susceptibility is not so obvious. A long-standing explanation has been that a blood-brain barrier develops with age, but the precise nature and location of this barrier has been obscure. A recent study (JOHNSON, 1964b) suggests that the difference between young and adult mice may reside in differences in the ability of peritoneal and tissue macrophages to spread herpes simplex virus infection. Although the cells of the central nervous system in the adult mouse are just as susceptible and will support the multiplication of herpes simplex virus to the same extent as the cells of the infant mouse, the ability of the macrophages to spread the disease to the central nervous system is decreased in the adult animal. It should be emphasized, however, that the macrophages may be only one factor playing a role in the spread of herpes simplex virus and that there may be additional factors involved in this process.

C. Dynamics of Development of Disease

1. Herpes Simplex Virus

a) Man

Herpes virus can be isolated from various organs of the body. SEIDENBERG (1941) and WENNER (1944) isolated herpes simplex virus from dermal lesions, as well as from the central nervous system, of patients with *eczema herpeticum*. Virus has also been isolated from the blood of adult patients and from children with generalized infection (BAKER et al., 1952; BECKER et al., 1963), as well as from patients with herpetic rhinitis (RUCHMAN and DODD, 1950) and herpes keratitis (LEOPOLD, 1965). Tissue and vesicle fluids from patients with *erythema multiforme* have also yielded virus (FOERSTER and SCOTT, 1958).

Information about the pathogenesis of infection in man is limited; most of the available knowledge about the development of herpes simplex virus infections is derived from experiments with animals, studies which have underlined the significance of the investigations with human beings. It is, however, known that herpes simplex virus enters the human body via the lips, mouth skin, conjunctival sac, or genitals, presumably multiplying at the site of entry. For example, primary herpetic stomatitis infection starts in the buccal mucosa and moves to neighboring cells and thence to skin areas by contaminated saliva.

b) Animals

Rabbits inoculated in the cornea of their eyes develop a keratitis that is similar to the same disease in man. In a recent study (ENGLE and STEWART, 1964), in which rabbit eyes were scarified and given about 10^5 TCID$_{50}$ doses, the ensuing herpes keratitis evolved as follows: Pinpoint dendritic lesions appeared when multiplication of the virus had reached a titer in the eye of about 10^4TCID$_{50}$, as measured in rabbit kidney cell cultures, whereas virus reached a maximum titer about 2 days after inoculation. The peak of damage to the cornea, involving more than half its area, did not occur until 5 to 7 days after infection. If the keratitis was left untreated, the rabbits developed fatal encephalitis within 4 to 5 days. BIEGELEISEN et al. (1957) found that following corneal inoculation of rabbits with herpes simplex virus, a viremia can be detected as early as 24 hours after inoculation and persists for as late as 132 hours after inoculation. Homogenates of brains, heart blood, spleen, heart, kidney, liver and lungs, yielded virus in these experiments. Rabbits will also develop encephalitis when inoculated peripherally with neurotropic strains and may even do so when they are placed in the same cages with rabbits inoculated on the cornea with herpes simplex virus. In this case, primary infection occurs in the mucous membranes of the mouth, nose or throat (GOODPASTURE, 1925b).

Guinea pigs are also susceptible to herpes simplex virus infection (VAN ROOYEN and RHODES, 1948; NICOLAU, 1948). Inoculation of herpes simplex virus into the footpads of guinea pigs causes the development of local lesions containing large amounts of virus, but viremia and generalization of the disease are not observed. On the other hand, inoculation of the virus into the blood stream produces a generalized type of herpes simplex infection in which the eyes, skin, vascular endothelium, adrenals, and brain are affected (PLATT, 1964).

The pathogenesis of herpes simplex virus in chick embryo was studied in detail by ANDERSON (1940). Virus adsorbed to intact, uninjured epithelium penetrates the epithelial cells and multiplies in these cells, developing the characteristic intranuclear inclusions and other cellular changes which are the same as those described in the section on Cytopathology. A hyperplasia of the epithelium occurs, producing the well-known pocks on the chorioallantoic membrane. The virus then spreads to contiguous epithelial cells and to other tissues. In general, the pathological process consists of proliferation, mild inflammation, necrosis, vesiculation, and desquamation. This is the pattern of pathogenesis not only after inoculation of the chorioallantois but also of cutaneous, pharyngeal, amniotic, and peritoneal infections that follow injection into the amniotic fluid. Virus spreads from the chorioallantois to the brain of the embryos which develop an encephalitis. Lesions are also found in the heart, liver, spleen, kidney, lung, and other organs. Inclusion bodies characteristic of herpes simplex virus may be observed in the endothelium of the blood vessels. Virus can be isolated from the blood-stream between 24 and 48 hours after inoculation depending on the source of the inoculum.

The mechanism of spread of herpes simplex virus from the periphery of an animal to its nervous system has been the subject of controversy. Three hypotheses have been formulated: (1) The virus invades the central nervous system via the bloodstream, (2) via the peripheral nerves that supply the inoculated area, or (3) via the tissue spaces and vessel sheaths of the nerves.

The first of these hypotheses was advanced by DOERR and VÖCHTING (1920) who had shown that disease of the central nervous system could be induced by intravenous inoculation of herpes simplex virus. However, GOODPASTURE and TEAGUE (1923) and GOODPASTURE (1925a) analyzed by histological means the pathogenesis of herpes simplex virus and came to the conclusion that the virus will reach the central nervous system, after multiplication of the virus at the site of inoculation, by way of the peripheral nerves that supply the inoculated area. The authors found that (1) when the cornea was inoculated, lesions in the sensory root of the fifth cranial nerve in the pons and medulla on the side inoculated could be observed; (2) when the virus was injected into the muscle of the hind leg of the rabbit, an acute myelitis resulted in the lumbar portion of the spinal cord; (3) when the virus was injected into the adrenal glands or the ovaries, an acute myelitis occurred at the level of the spinal cord where the sympathetic fibers of these organs enter. GOODPASTURE (1925a) concluded from his experiments that the axis-cylinder of the peripheral nerves serve as the pathways for the movement of herpes simplex virus into the central nervous system, a movement that occurs by continued multiplication of the virus. (The concept of the replication of herpes simplex virus in the axons is difficult to accept in view of the fact that infectious virus is assembled within the nuclei of infected cells.) MARINESCO and DRAGANESCO (1923), basing themselves on analogous data, concluded that although movement along the axons does occur, the actual pathway to the central nervous system is via the tissue spaces and vessel sheaths of the nerves and not the axons themselves.

This controversy was resumed more than twenty five years later when FIELD (1952) re-analyzed in rabbits the mode of transmission of the virus from the cornea and from the masseter muscle to the central nervous system and reported that his results were not consistent with a centripetal spread of the virus via the axons; he concluded that the lymphatic system plays the essential role in the mechanism of ascent.

The studies on the mode of spread of herpes simplex virus described above were based primarily on pathological and clinical criteria and on relatively crude methods of titrations of virus. In recent years, the problem of the pathogenesis of herpes simplex virus encephalitis has been re-investigated by modern methods, and it appears that virus introduced into the animal peripherally reaches the central nervous system via hematogenous or neural routes, depending upon the route of inoculation.

WILDY (1954) was the first to present unequivocal evidence that the virus can spread centripetally to the central nervous system. Virus was inoculated into the rear footpad of 5-week-old mice and the virus titer in different organs

Table 6. *Transmission of Herpes Simplex Virus[1] during Pathogenesis of Encephalitis in Newborn Mice*

Route of Inoculation	LD$_{50}$ (PFU)	Distribution and movement of virus
Intracerebral[2]	3	No significant extraneural multiplication. Virus antigen detectable only within CNS[5]. Dispersion of virus via CSF[5] with initial multiplication in mesenchymal cells of meninges and ectodermal lining of ventricles. Infection spreads directly into underlying CNS involving neurons and glial cells.
Intraperitoneal[2]	14	Viremia develops within 5 hours and persists until death. Initial growth of virus in free peritoneal macrophages, then along serosal surfaces, and within parenchyma of liver and spleen. Infection of CNS blood-borne, with virus antigen appearing first around small cerebral vessels.
Subcutaneous[3]	1.4×10^4	Infection of a few subcutaneous cells, most likely histiocytes, and the endoneural cells of subcutaneous nerve fibers. No viremia or visceral infection. Virus reaches CNS by centripetal infection of endoneural cells only.
Intranasal[4]	1.4×10^4	Virus reaches CNS via multiple neural pathways and via blood. Direct invasion of subarachnoid space with dispersions of virus in CSF similar to spread after intracerebral inoculation, infection of cells along nerves (both olfactory and trigeminal) similar to spread after subcutaneous inoculation, and hematogenous infection similar to spread after intraperitoneal inoculation.

From JOHNSON (1964).

[1] HFEM strain.
[2] 100 LD$_{50}$ injected.
[3] 5×10^4 PFU injected.
[4] Droplet containing 5×10^4 PFU inhaled.
[5] CNS, central nervous system; CSF, cerebrospinal fluid.

was determined. Despite posterior paralysis there was no viremia and neural spread of the virus to the central nervous system seems therefore to have occurred. In more recent experiments, WILDY (1967) found that conditions can be created in which invasion of the central nervous system occurs in mice inoculated intradermally with herpes virus. In these animals, invasion of the central nervous system was prevented by the interruption of the local peripheral nerve although infectious virus was present in the blood. These experiments were, however, performed in 5-week-old mice which do not develop nervous symptoms after peripheral inoculation with herpes virus, unless they have been previously traumatized; invasion of the central nervous system via hematogenous routes may, therefore, occur in naturally more sensitive animals.

In a very careful analysis of the course of spread of herpes simplex virus to the central nervous system, JOHNSON (1964a) made use of the sensitive technique of fluorescent antibody staining, as well as of histological and virus titration methods. Suckling mice were used in these studies, because encephalitis normally develops in these animals after peripheral inoculation, a response not found in adult mice. The results of these experiments show rather convincingly that herpes simplex virus does enter the central nervous system of suckling mice via either the hematogenous and the neural routes, depending upon the site of inoculation (see Table 6). These studies also demonstrated that the centripetal movement of herpes simplex virus is by way of ascending infection of the neural cells, not by way of the axons. JOHNSON's experiments showed also that after intranasal inoculation, there are multiple ascending pathways of the virus to the central nervous system, as well as a blood borne infection, thus clarifying the controversy engendered by the conflicting results obtained from many studies on this subject (BURNET and LUSH, 1939b; LEVADITI et al., 1935; KING, 1940; SLAVIN and BERRY, 1943).

2. Pseudorabies Virus

In swine, infection with pseudorabies virus is usually nonfatal, and the animals pass through a mild febrile disease. In a study of naturally infected swine, MAŠIĆ et al. (1965) showed that pseudorabies virus multiplies primarily in the tonsils and appears to spread via the bloodstream to the central nervous system, lungs, and gravid uterus in which pathological changes can be observed.

The distribution of pseudorabies virus was followed in pigs after intranasal inoculation (McFERRAN and Dow, 1965). Under these conditions, the primary site of virus multiplication is the respiratory tract: virus can be isolated from the nasal, pharyngeal, and tracheal mucosa by about 24 hours after infection; virus can also be detected in the lymph nodes draining these sites. Excretion of virus continues from these areas for about 10 days but not thereafter. Virus appears to spread from the respiratory tract (within 48 to 72 hours) by way of the olfactory nerves to the olfactory bulbs or by the glossopharyngeal nerve from the pharynx to the nucleus solitarus in the medulla; both routes are sometimes used in the same animals. Another pathway, the trigeminal nerve to the pons and medulla, has been found in other animals. After reaching the brain, there is a relatively rapid centrifugal spread of the virus from the point of entry. The virus multiplies in the brain to a limited degree only. The central nervous system of the swine seems to be resistant to the effect of pseudorabies virus and in most cases the animals survive infection. After about 8 to 10 days there is a quick disappearance of detectable virus from the central nervous system. It is of interest to note that at the time the virus is disappearing from the brain, neutralizing antibody begins to appear in the blood (McFERRAN and Dow, 1965). However, pseudorabies virus is always fatal when inoculated intracerebrally into swine and virus spreads rapidly from the site of inoculation where multiplication first occurs (HURST, 1933).

Cattle, which are among the most susceptible of the domestic animals to pseudorabies virus, exhibit neurological signs and invariably die. After infection by any route (intranasal, subcutaneous, and intramuscular) virus moves centripetally from the peripheral nerves to the central nervous system and then centrifugally through the central nervous system (MCFERRAN and DOW, 1964b). Virus cannot be isolated from the blood of the animals, and the absence of virus from the cerebro-spinal fluid supports the view that in cattle, at least, pseudorabies virus appears to be strictly neurotropic.

Many laboratory animals are highly susceptible to the virus. One of the characteristic manifestations of infection with pseudorabies virus in some of these animals is the itching that occurs at the site of inoculation when the virus reaches the appropriate spinal root ganglion. The pathogenesis of the disease in laboratory animals does depend on the route of inoculation (HURST, 1933; OLANDER et al., 1966) and, as in the case of herpes simplex virus, there has been some controversy about the pathway of spread from peripheral areas to the central nervous system (hematogenous or neural). It appears likely that both modes of transmission are operative.

Among laboratory animals, the rabbit is, perhaps, the most sensitive to pseudorabies virus. Following intramuscular, intradermal, and subcutaneous inoculation, pseudorabies virus reaches the central nervous system via the peripheral nerves. After intracerebral inoculation, the virus passes in the reverse direction with a centrifugal spread to the nerve axis. Virus can be found in the bloodstream, and, in fact, very small inocula are required to produce the disease by intravenous inoculation; this route of inoculation results in the formation of foci of virus multiplication in various organs. From these organs, the virus ascends the peripheral nerves to reach the central nervous system, the precise symptomatology differing depending on whether the spinal cord or medulla is reached first (HURST, 1934).

Although virus can reach the central nervous system after subcutaneous inoculation of rabbit feet which have been denervated (the sciatic nerve was excised), HURST (1934) considered the spread to be indirect; that is, virus moves via the bloodstream to various organs (spleen, liver, adrenals, etc.) where the virus multiplies and then moves to the central nervous system via peripheral nerves. REMLINGER and BAILLY (1933) concluded, however, from similar experiments that pseudorabies virus reaches the central nervous system via the bloodstream and not via the peripheral nerves. Although most of the evidence to date suggests that pseudorabies virus has a strong predilection for nervous tissue and probably does move to the central nervous system by way of peripheral nerves, there is no analytical study available at the present time which uses modern techniques to preclude the possibility that virus may also reach the central nervous system by way of the bloodstream.

Mice are also highly susceptible to pseudorabies virus (KING, 1940). Observations with these animals indicate that virus multiplies at the local site of inoculation, invades the local nerve, and then proceeds to the central nervous system via this pathway.

Monkeys *(Macaca mulatta)* are susceptible to pseudorabies virus only when these animals are inoculated by the intracerebral, intrasciatic, or intracisternal routes, indicating a strict predeliction for nervous tissue (HURST, 1936). Large doses of virus introduced intradermally, intramuscularly, or intravenously do not produce infection in the monkeys. This would indicate that the virus does not multiply sufficiently at the site of inoculation to reach the peripheral nerves from which the virus would ascend into the central nervous system. However, inoculation directly into the sciatic nerve suffices to cause the virus to move to the central nervous system. Thus, the nervous system of monkeys is highly susceptible to pseudorabies virus, but if virus does not come in contact with the nerves, infection does not ensue. The resistance of the monkeys is to be contrasted with the resistance of swine to pseudorabies virus. In swine the virus reaches the brain after peripheral inoculation but the virus replicates in the central nervous system to a limited degree only.

In the chick embryo, virus multiplies in the chorioallantoic membrane, as well as within the central nervous system (BANG, 1942). Since the bloodstream is the only avenue to the embryo from the chorioallantoic membrane, it is obvious that the virus must reach the embryo via the blood. However, it is not clear from this study whether virus reaches the central nervous system via the bloodstream or whether virus multiplies first at some site in the embryo and then ascends the peripheral nerves to the central nervous system.

X. Variation
A. Virulence and Cytopathogenicity

The classic method of isolation of viruses from nature by the inoculation of laboratory animals or, in more recent years, of cell cultures, constitutes an important step in the selection of variants. Frequently, the newly-isolated strains will multiply with difficulty on first passage in their new host and will grow rapidly only after a certain number of passages. This is an example of population genetics, in which variants capable of multiplying in cells of a new host are being selected by continuous passage in this host. This sequence of events occurs with all viruses, including herpes simplex virus and pseudorabies virus.

A number of variants of herpes simplex and pseudorabies virus has been described. During a study of the pathogenesis of herpes simplex virus in the chick embryo, ANDERSON (1940) noted that while 12- or 13-day-old chick embryos inoculated with the classic HF strain of this virus usually survived about seven days, embryos inoculated with virus after it had been passed 125 times in chick embryos usually died about 96 hours after infection. Another example of the effect of passaging a virus strain in laboratory animals is provided by BESWICK (1958). Newborn mice inoculated intraperitoneally with a newly-isolated strain of herpes simplex virus exhibited an ascending myelitis followed by paralysis but only mild lesions in the peritoneal cavity. After this strain had been passed in rabbits, suckling mice and chick embryos, it caused fewer lesions in the central nervous system and paralysis was no longer observed; instead, the organs within the peritoneal cavity began to show lesions of increasing severity and extent. NOJIMA (1960) has also provided an example for this kind of effect; he found that a freshly isolated strain of herpes simplex virus lost its pathogenicity for baby mice, when infected intraperitoneally, after about 25 passages in chick embryos.

Selection of mutants has also been reported for pseudorabies virus. A mutant of pseudorabies virus with an altered virulence was isolated by repeated passage of the virus in pigeons. This mutant showed increased virulence for pigeons, animals not normally susceptible to pseudorabies virus; the virulence of the mutant virus for rabbits and mice was, on the other hand, decreased (TONEVA, 1961). The cultivation of pseudorabies virus on the chorioallantoic membrane of chick embryos (GLOVER, 1939) or in chick embryo cells *in vitro* (IVÁNOVICS et al., 1955b) caused the loss of, or at least a diminution in, the appearance of pruritus at the site of inoculation in rabbits or mice.

Attenuated strains of pseudorabies virus have been isolated after many successive, usually hundreds of passages in chick embryo cultures *in vitro*. Generally, these attenuated strains show an absence of pruritus in rabbits and appear to have lost their virulence for swine, which develop immunity to the disease after being inoculated with the attenuated strains. In some cases, these strains also show reduced virulence for cattle and sheep (MAYER and ŠKODA, 1962; BARTHA and KOJNOK, 1962; ŠKODA, 1962; ŽUFFA, 1963; ŠKODA et al., 1964a and b; ŠKODA and JAMARICHOVÁ, 1965).

Since variants in pathogenicity can be isolated easily from a given strain, it is not surprising that different strains will vary among themselves in this respect. CHU and WARREN (1960) have shown that 4 strains of herpes simplex virus separately isolated from nature by cultivation in rabbit kidney cells exhibited marked differences with respect to their cytopathic effects and in their virulence for chick embryos, mice and, other laboratory animals.

The fact that passage of a virus strain in a normally nonsusceptible host will eventually yield virus with altered properties indicates that the original virus population is mixed and probably contains viruses with different degrees of virulence for the various hosts. That the variants are present in relatively large numbers in the original virus population is demonstrated by the fact that this type of variant can be isolated without using enrichment procedures. For example, KOHLHAGE and SIEGERT (1962) isolated by the terminal dilution technique from the JES strain of herpes simplex virus two variants differing in virulence. One of the variants was less virulent than the other in producing keratitis in the rabbit eye and was also less virulent for mice inoculated intracerebrally. These two variants caused different types of cytopathic effects in HeLa cell cultures: one formed giant cells and the other, flat syncytia with many nuclei. Otherwise, the two variants were indistinguishable. RAPP (1963) isolated a number of variants from plaques formed under agar. A relation between the type of cytopathic effect produced by the virus mutant and virulence was also found for these variants. Whereas large plaque-formers generally produced keratitis on the cornea of rabbits and showed approximately the same neuro-virulence for weanling mice as the parent strain, most small plaque-formers did not produce keratitis in rabbits and were only about 1% as virulent as the parental virus strain for weanling mice.

Mutants of herpes simplex virus which produce different cytopathic effects in cell culture have been isolated repeatedly. The differences between these mutants with respect to a number of other properties vary in degree. Thus, SCOTT and his associates (GRAY et al., 1958; SCOTT and McLEOD, 1959; SCOTT et al., 1961) have isolated two mutants of herpes simplex virus from the same virus stock which produced two different kinds of cytopathic effect. One produced rounded balloon cells and the other, syncytial masses; the two strains were otherwise identical. WHEELER (1964) also isolated two variants of herpes simplex virus, one of which produced syncytia and the other, small giant cells in monolayer cultures of HeLa cells; these two mutants, however, differed slightly with respect to their antigenic structure.

Two variants of herpes simplex virus which differed from each other in several characteristics have been isolated (HOGGAN and ROIZMAN, 1959; HOGGAN et al., 1961). These mutants differed in the size of their plaques, in the type of cytopathic effect they produced, and appeared to have somewhat different surface properties. Not only were differences revealed between these two variants of viruses by cross-neutralization tests, but also in their elution pattern from Brushite columns of calcium phosphate. Furthermore, these 2 mutants appeared to have different buoyant densities in cesium chloride (ROIZMAN and ROANE, 1961 and 1963).

A difference in the surface properties of two variants of herpes simplex virus differing in the type of cytopathic effect they produced in cell culture has also been reported by KOHLHAGE and SIEGERT (1962) and KOHLHAGE (1964). In this case, although the two variants could not be differentiated on the basis of antigenicity, they did show differences in elution from columns of ECTEOLA, as well as in their buoyant density. These strains also showed differences in neurovirulence.

The isolation of mutants of herpes simplex virus that produce different kinds of degeneration in cell culture and that appear to differ in their physical and chemical properties has been described for other virus strains, as well (FALKE, 1964 and 1965; NII and KAMAHORA, 1961; NII, 1961).

Mutants of pseudorabies virus differing in their cytopathic effects have also been reported. TOKUMARU (1957) isolated two variants of pseudorabies virus from monkey kidney cells which exhibited different cytopathic features: the G strain produced small plaques and caused cell rounding, whereas the L strain produced large plaques and formed cytolytic giant cells. In contrast to the L strain, the G strain either produced a weak pruritus or none at all after inoculation into rats. Another small plaque variant of pseudorabies virus that lost its ability to produce pruritus in rabbits and also had a reduced virulence for rabbits and none at all for pigs and sheep has been isolated from plaques on pig kidney cells (BARTHA, 1961; BARTHA and KOJNOK, 1962); these properties have persisted for at least 70 passages in cell cultures.

B. Conditional Lethal Mutants

Conditional lethal mutants of herpes simplex virus have recently been isolated (AURELIAN and ROIZMAN, 1964; ROIZMAN and AURELIAN, 1965; AURELIAN and ROIZMAN, 1965; ROIZMAN, 1965). While these mutants (MPdk⁻) can grow normally in one host (HEp-2 cells), they have a genetic defect that does not allow them to multiply in another. Thus, this mutant fails to produce infectious progeny in dog kidney cells which, however, do form viral antigen, interferon, and small amounts of viral DNA. Although viral particles are not formed in these cells, the cells exhibit cytopathic changes after infection. It appears that in dog kidney cells, one or more structural constituents of the MPdk⁻ virion are either not made or are non-functional. Continued propagation of MPdk⁻ in dog kidney cells yield mutants that produce small (MPdk⁺sp) and large (MPdk⁺lp) plaques in human, as well as in canine, cells. The two mutants, MPdk⁺sp and MPdk⁺lp, differ from the original MPdk⁻ strain with respect to plaque morphology in human cells, buoyant density in cesium chloride density gradients, stability at 40°C, and reactivity with antiserum prepared against MPdk⁻ virus.

C. Drug-resistant Mutants

Herpes keratitis is one of the first viral diseases to have been controlled by chemotherapy. However, one of the practical problems in the chemotherapy of diseases caused by herpes simplex virus is the frequent appearance of virus mutants that are resistant to antiviral agents. Thus, cultures infected with herpes simplex virus and incubated in the presence of IUdR or BUdR eventually yield virus that is able to replicate in the presence of very high doses of these drugs (BUTHALA, 1964; DUBBS and KIT, 1964; EGGERS and TAMM, 1966). Mutants resistant to Ara-C have, however, not as yet been isolated.

DUBBS and KIT (1964) have isolated mutants of herpes simplex virus that are unable to induce an increase in the activity of thymidine kinase. (The activity of this enzyme is increased by infection of cells with wild type herpes simplex virus.) These mutants were isolated by growing the virus in mouse fibroblasts lacking thymidine kinase activity (strain LMTK⁻) in the presence of BUdR. However, the mutants will also multiply to some extent in normal mouse fibroblast cells treated with BUdR, and it seems, therefore, that the mutants that appear in IUdR and BUdR treated cultures may lack the ability to induce thymidine kinase in the infected cells. In addition to mutants that always induce only very low levels of activity of thymidine kinase in LMTK⁻ cells, "leaky" mutants have also been isolated. These "leaky" mutants will induce an increase in the activity of thymidine kinase when the infected cells are grown at 31°C, but only a slight increase in activity will be observed when the cells are grown at 37°C (DUBBS and KIT, 1965).

XI. Immunity
A. Active Immunization
1. Immunity Resulting from Natural Infection

In nature, man is constantly being infected with herpes simplex virus, and in most instances, individuals survive the diseases caused by this virus, diseases which are frequently subclinical. This is a natural immunization and such individuals usually possess high titers of virus-specific antibody. Thus, infectious herpes simplex virus is a good antigen and will produce relatively high amounts of antibody. This is further demonstrated by the fact that convalescent sera of laboratory animals inoculated with virus and that survive infection possess antibody against herpes simplex virus.

Although herpes simplex virus generally only causes mild febrile diseases in man (see below), it may be potentially dangerous; it is desirable therefore to try to develop vaccines of attenuated or killed virus.

Naturally acquired immunity to pseudorabies virus occurs also in swine. However, epidemics of pseudorabies virus infection in swine, as well as in other domestic animals, have been a severe economic problem and attempts to develop vaccines against this disease have also been made.

2. Immunization with Attenuated Virus

Little effort has been expended in attempting to produce attenuated strains of herpes simplex virus for the purpose of immunization. Attenuated strains of pseudorabies virus have, however, been utilized for this purpose.

A variant of pseudorabies virus isolated in pig kidney cells that exhibited decreased virulence for rabbits and none for domestic animals has been used as an attenuated vaccine. The variant was propagated in monolayer cultures of chick embryo cells and the culture fluids were used, as such, as the vaccine. Fourteen pigs were inoculated once and seven pigs were inoculated twice with this virus; neutralizing antibodies could be detected only in the blood of the latter group of animals. Nevertheless, all 21 immunized pigs resisted a challenge infection with virulent pseudorabies virus, whereas all control animals (8 pigs) succumbed to the inoculation.

This attenuated virus strain also produced some immunity in sheep. The vaccine was injected into 14 sheep; of this number, 2 died and 12 survived challenge with virulent virus given intramuscularly (BARTHA, 1961; BARTHA and KOJNOK, 1962; BARÓCASAI and TANCZER, 1962).

By repeated passage of pseudorabies virus in chick embryo cells, an attenuated strain (BUK) was obtained that proved effective in the immunization of two month old calves. Doses of approximately 10^5 to 10^8 $TCID_{50}$ of the attenuated strain induced the formation in about 2 to 5 weeks of neutralizing antibodies in the serum that reached titers of 1:4 to 1:64 against 100 to 1,000 $TCID_{50}$ of virus. These calves did not succumb to an intramuscular inoculation of virulent virus; this inoculation further increased the titer of neutralizing antibody present in the sera of these animals (ŠKODA, 1962; ŠKODA et al., 1964a). The same strain was also tested as a vaccine in suckling pigs, weanlings, young pigs and sows. It was found that the attenuated virus was successful in inducing the formation of neutralizing antibodies in these animals and that they resisted challenge with virulent virus. The development of neutralizing antibodies was, however, slow and up to seven weeks were required to reach significant titers. The titers obtained were not as high as those produced after the natural disease in pigs; however, revaccination of the animals increased the titers to satisfactory levels (ŠKODA et al., 1964b). When this vaccine was tested under field conditions with large numbers of pigs, the vaccine proved highly successful (ŠKODA et al., 1966).

Other attenuated vaccines, which were also produced by repeated passage in cells cultivated *in vitro*, have been reported to protect pigs, sheep, and calves against inoculation with virulent pseudorabies virus (ŽUFFA, 1963; BALDELLI et al., 1964).

3. Immunization with Killed Virus

Early efforts to produce a killed virus vaccine consisted of emulsifying tissues from infected animals (usually brains of rabbits and guinea pigs) and treating them with phenol, formalin, or heat. Inoculation of these vaccines into man appeared to produce a certain degree of immunity against herpes simplex virus, as measured by a decrease in the severity of the disease (HOLDEN, 1932; MARTIN and CANEJA, 1933; BRAIN, 1936; FRANK, 1938). These vaccines also induced the formation of antibody in animals (URBAIN and SCHAEFFER, 1929; BEDSON, 1931; KANAZAWA, 1938; BURNET and LUSH, 1939b). However, in addition to the fact that the immunity induced in man by these vaccines was of a questionable nature, they were prepared from nervous tissue and were therefore dangerous.

Later attempts to produce a vaccine, chiefly with allantoic fluids from infected embryonated eggs (a more desirable source of herpes simplex virus than the ones used in the earlier experiments) inactivated by treatment with formalin or ultraviolet light irradiation led to the view that inactivated vaccines of herpes simplex virus are not effective as immunizing agents (ANDERSON et al., 1950; JAWETZ et al., 1951 and 1955). However, the failure of these attempts to produce a vaccine with this material was probably due to the low concentrations of virus, as well as to the presence of a great deal of extraneous protein. In addition, the inactivation of the virus may have been excessive, so that not only was virus infectivity lost but antigenicity, as well.

Some of these problems have been overcome in recent years by the use of cells cultured *in vitro*, from which preparations with high titers of virus and which are relatively free of cell material can be obtained, thus making purification of the virus simpler.

Using these methods, some success has been achieved in the production of inactivated herpes vaccines effective in immunizing mice and guinea pigs.

Herpes simplex virus cultivated in rabbit kidney cells *in vitro* and inactivated by irradiation with ultraviolet light was injected intravenously and intraperitoneally into mice. Most of the infected animals became immune and survived intracerebral challenge with 1,000 ID_{50} doses of infectious virus. The immunized mice also possessed neutralizing antibody (ANDERSON and KILBOURNE, 1961a). The successful production of a herpes simplex virus vaccine prepared from virus cultivated on sheep embryo kidney cells and inactivated by irradiation with ultraviolet light has also been reported (LÉPINE et al., 1964). A vaccine prepared by treatment with formalin of herpes simplex virus grown in rabbit kidney cells *in vitro* that induces the formation of neutralizing antibodies in animals has also been produced; it was highly potent in guinea pigs and in mice and the infected animals resisted intracerebral challenge with high doses of virulent virus (CHU and WARREN, 1960).

The production of herpes simplex virus vaccines effective in immunizing animals sparked efforts to manufacture a killed-virus vaccine for the control of diseases caused by the virus in human beings. This vaccine is essential in order to prevent the possibility of death resulting from a primary infection or blindness resulting from recurrent infections of the cornea. Herpes simplex virus cultivated in rabbit kidney cell cultures was clarified by filtration and then inactivated by treatment with formalin and incubation at 37°C (CHAPIN et al., 1962; KERN and SCHIFF, 1964; HULL and PECK, 1967). Although these vaccines did produce neutralizing antibody after inoculation of guinea pigs and rabbits, they had little or no effect in producing antibodies in human beings, even after 10 weekly subcutaneous doses. However, these vaccines appeared to be of some benefit to patients suffering from recurrent herpes simplex virus infections, as well as from keratitis of the cornea. After treatment of these patients with the vaccines, there semed to be a lessening of the severity of the disease and, in some cases, complete remission. Similar results have been reported using virus preparations inactivated by ultraviolet light (LÉPINE et al., 1964; HENOCQ et al., 1964). It should be emphasized, however, that the estimation of the value of a vaccine to a patient is subjective and difficult to evaluate. Furthermore, there may be some dangers to the use of a herpes simplex virus vaccine. Thus, a patient who did not have an earlier history of clinical herpes came down with a case of genital herpes after vaccination; another patient had an exacerbation of acute herpes keratitis (CHAPIN et al., 1962).

Many attempts have been made in the past to produce inactivated pseudorabies virus vaccine, particularly in Eastern Europe where killed-virus vaccines have been tested repeatedly but without success (MANNINGER and MÓCZY, 1959). However, HULL and PECK (1967) have prepared a vaccine by filtration and treatment of formalin at 37°C that was antigenic for rabbits and mice and appeared to be effective in protecting 6 month old calves. Four calves given multiple doses of this vaccine developed by 6 weeks after the last dose an increase in antibody titer and survived challenge with virulent virus; the controls succumbed to infection. These results are encouraging and indicate that in addition to the attenuated vaccine described above, an effective killed-virus vaccine can also probably be produced.

B. Passive Immunization

It has been known for many years that animals given hyperimmune serum against herpes simplex virus will be protected against challenge with virulent virus (BEDSON and CRAWFORD, 1927; ANDERVONT, 1929b; BURNET and LUSH, 1939a; ANDERSON, 1940; BERRY and SLAVIN, 1943; EVANS et al., 1946). In general, the shorter the interval between the injection of the antiserum and of the virus, the better the chance of survival of the animals. Passive immunity also exists in neonatal animals by virtue of the passage of antibody from immunized mothers to the embryos; this passive immunity lasts for varying periods of time, depending upon the species tested.

There have been conflicting reports about the efficacy of the injection of human γ-globulin into human beings as a means of preventing or ameliorating infections caused by herpes simplex virus. In one clinical observation, a 17-year-old girl suffering from eczema herpeticum appeared to have benefited from injections of human γ-globulin (RUPPE et al., 1957). On the other hand, failures have been reported on the ability of γ-globulin to prevent disease in newborn infants (SCOTT, 1967). There have been no well-controlled studies on the use of γ-globulin as a means of passive immunization of individuals against herpes virus-induced diseases, and until these studies are carried out, the value of γ-globulin as a preventive agent remains an open question.

Piglets of immune mothers are usually resistant to challenge with pseudorabies virus, and it has been clearly demonstrated that this resistance is due to
the passage of antibody from the sows to their offspring via colostrum and
milk (KOJNOK and SURJAN, 1963; ŠKODA et al., 1963; AKKERMANNS, 1963;
ŽUFFA, 1964; ŠKODA et al., 1964b and 1966). During the first few hours after
delivery, a large quantity of neutralizing antibody is found in the colostrum,
the amount being directly proportional to the amount present in the serum. By
the end of about 24 hours *post partum*, there is a decrease in the concentration
of antibody in the colostrum and by 7 to 10 days, antibody is no longer detectable. The quantitative level of neutralizing antibody in the serum of the
piglets is dependent upon the amount of antibody present in the colostrum and
milk. There is an initial high level of neutralizing antibody in the piglet serum
which decreases gradually, so that by 45 to 50 days after birth, there is practically
none left (KOJNOK and SURJAN, 1963). Piglets with antibodies in their serum
resist challenge with pseudorabies virus.

Passive experimental immunization against pseudorabies virus infection has
also been achieved: Rabbits and suckling pigs given hyperimmune serum subcutaneously, intraperitoneally, or intravenously survive infection with virulent
pseudorabies virus. Furthermore, in a field test in large pig farms in which the
pigs were infected with pseudorabies virus (as determined by autopsy) only
63 out of 923 (6.7%) suckling pigs given hyperimmune serum died, whereas
229 out of 752 (30.4%) untreated controls died, indicating that the antiserum
was effective in controlling the epizootic (KOJNOK and GRÉCZI, 1957).

Similar results were also obtained by LUKASHOV and NIKITIN (1958) who
found that 10% γ-globulin from immune sera given to pigs 24 hours before
inoculation with virulent virus protects the animals against infection and that
γ-globulin may also be used therapeutically.

C. Interference and Interferon

The ability of one virus, active or inactive, to prevent the replication of a
second related or unrelated virus was recognized early as an important biological
phenomenon. Not only was this phenomenon of widespread theoretical interest
but it had medical significance, as well. Many viruses were soon tested for their
capacity to interfere with the replication of another, and among them was herpes
simplex virus.

Thus, for example, herpes simplex virus was found to interfere with the
replication of rabies, an unrelated virus (LEVADITI, 1942). More recently, BARSKI
(1963) found that hamsters inoculated intraperitoneally with herpes simplex
virus will resist almost completely most of the pathological consequences of infection with polyoma virus inoculated by the same route 24 to 48 hours later. The
nature of this interference is not known, although, on the basis of temporal considerations, the role of specific antibody could be ruled out.

In addition to interference between herpes simplex and unrelated viruses,
interference has been demonstrated between strains of herpes simplex virus
itself. Perhaps one of the most interesting studies on virus interference involves
the classic "Konkurrenz-Phänomen" of MAGRASSI (MAGRASSI, 1935 and 1936;
DOERR and KON, 1937; DOERR and SEIDENBERG, 1937; HALLAUER, 1937). This

is an example of two strains of herpes simplex virus, one encephalitogenic and one nonencephalitogenic, that interfere with each other. Thus, when the nonencephalitogenic strain is inoculated into the cornea of a rabbit, it travels by way of the trigeminal nerve to the brain and prevents the development of encephalitis after the intracerebral inoculation of a virulent encephalitogenic strain a few days later. Actually, a virulent encephalitogenic strain can also be used for the primary inoculation of the cornea; the second, intracerebral injection of the virulent strain not only fails to produce encephalitis itself, but prevents the development of encephalitis by the first virus. Both viruses disappear eventually from the brain. Although this phenomenon has been considered a classic example of virus interference, it has not been adequately explained. In fact, the role of local, specific immunity has not been entirely ruled out (SCHLESINGER, 1959).

Since the development of cell culture methods, there have been many examples of interference *in vitro*, and in several instances, the interference appeared to have occurred without the intervention of interferon. This type of interference has been demonstrated in cell culture between 2 mutants of herpes simplex virus (ROIZMAN, 1965). Variants of pseudorabies virus have also been found to interfere with one another in cell culture but it is not known whether interferon was involved (IVÁNOVICS et al., 1955a). A recent observation by VAN DER NOORDAA et al. (1966) is of particular interest: hamster and human cells transformed by SV40 resisted infection with herpes simplex virus, a resistance that could not be ascribed to interferon but possibly to the fact that both viruses are produced in the cell nucleus.

Interference is not the invariable consequence of infection of a host with two viruses; on the contrary, dual infection of cells with herpes simplex and a second virus has been reported on several occasions. For example, infection of cells with fowlpox virus does not prevent the multiplication of herpes simplex virus and the cells support the growth of both viruses (ANDERSON, 1942). There are additional instances in which cells, infected first by herpes simplex virus and then by vaccinia, fowlpox, or rabies allow the growth of both viruses (ANDERSON, 1942; SYVERTON and BERRY, 1947; LEVADITI and REINIE, 1940).

Despite extensive studies, the mechanism of interference remained elusive, and since interference was a laboratory model with no obvious practical application, it tended to be regarded as nothing more than a curiosity, a once exciting phase in the history of experimental virology. However, the discovery of interferon by ISAACS and LINDENMANN (1957) renewed interest in the phenomenon.

Interferon, a protein that is produced by cells following inoculation with active or inactive viruses, as well as by a variety of non-viral substances (BARON and LEVY, 1966), interferes with the multiplication of many different viruses.

The interferon produced by herpes simplex virus in chick embryo cells is a protein of low molecular weight (about 36,000) that has the same properties as interferon produced in these cells by other agents: sensitivity to trypsin, relative heat stability (70°C), stability over a wide range of pH (1 to 11), and an isoelectric point around pH 7. Biologically, like all interferon preparations studied, this interferon is highly species specific but not virus specific; vesicular stomatitis virus is inhibited by the interferon produced by chick embryo cells infected with herpes simplex virus in chick embryo cells but not in mouse embryo cells, grivet kidney cells, bovine kidney cells or rabbit kidney cells (LAMPSON et al., 1965).

Interferon is produced in herpes simplex virus-infected cultures in which the virus multiplies, as well as in infected cultures which do not produce infectious virus. Thus, interferon is produced by chick embryo cultures that undergo cytopathic changes and cell lysis after infection with active herpes simplex virus; this interferon is active against Sindbis and vesicular stomatitis viruses (LAMPSON et al., 1965). Interferon is also produced in infected dog kidney cells in which infectious herpes simplex virus is not formed (AURELIAN and ROIZMAN, 1964). Furthermore, in certain cases, the production of interferon seems to be inversely related to the ability of the virus to replicate productively. Infection of dog kidney cells with the host-range mutant, MPdk$^+$, yields infectious progeny but no interferon (AURELIAN and ROIZMAN, 1965); this mutant also inhibits the synthesis of host cell RNA. The mutant, MPdk$^-$, which abortively infects dog-kidney cells and does not interfere with host cell RNA synthesis, does produce interferon.

Noninfectious herpes simplex virus also induces readily the formation of interferon. Thus, herpes simplex virus inactivated by ultraviolet light will produce in chick embryos interferon which is released into the allantoic fluid and which is effective to the same degree against herpes simplex virus and vaccinia virus (FRUITSTONE et al., 1964).

The ability of a continuous line of mouse embryo cell culture persistently infected with polyoma virus to resist challenge inoculation with low multiplicities of infection of herpes simplex virus has been found to depend upon the production of interferon by the challenge virus (GLASGOW and HABEL, 1963). Protection of the persistently infected culture was, however, not dependent solely upon the interferon produced by herpes simplex virus but upon the combined effect of this interferon together with that induced by polyoma virus itself. Either of these interferons acting alone was ineffective in protecting the cultures.

Interferon has also been produced in rabbits (FORCE et al., 1965). The interferon produced in the dermis of the rabbit suppressed the replication of vesicular stomatitis in cell culture and possessed the same properties as all other interferons.

The first experiments on the effect of interferon (produced by ultraviolet light irradiated-influenza virus in whole chorioallantoic membranes *in vitro*) on the multiplication of herpes simplex virus were equivocal; although a comparison of the growth of herpes simplex virus on the chorioallantoic membrane of embryonated eggs treated with interferon prior to inoculation and the untreated control revealed no significant differences in the pock count, these results were uncertain because there was a considerable variation in the pock counts from egg to egg (ISAACS et al., 1958). However, a virus inhibitory fluid, probably interferon, obtained from cultures infected with a chick embryo-adapted strain of poliovirus, seemed to have a slight but definite inhibitory effect on the multiplication of herpes simplex virus (HO and ENDERS, 1959); ISAACS (1961) later found that herpes simplex virus could be inhibited by large doses of interferon. An interferon produced by ultraviolet light irradiated vaccinia virus was far more effective than influenza interferon in inhibiting herpes simplex virus (GLASGOW and HABEL, 1962). A culture carrying polyoma virus also appears to have produced interferon capable of inhibiting herpes simplex virus (BARSKI and CORNE-FERT, 1962). The differences in results obtained with different interferon prep-arations are probably quantitative in nature and it seems that herpes simplex virus requires relatively large doses of interferon to inhibit its growth.

The effect of interferon (produced in chick embryo cells with western equine encephalomyelitis virus) on the replication of herpes simplex virus has been analyzed in detail (BROWN, 1966). Although this interferon preparation was more effective against western equine encephalomyelitis virus (which contains RNA) by a factor of 100, it was still quite inhibitory to herpes simplex virus. The protective effect of interferon was expressed only if it was added prior to infection, and was lost gradually as the interval between the addition of interferon and virus inoculation was lengthened. The loss in the capacity of the cells to produce infectious virus was greatest for the first 6 hours after the addition of interferon and declined thereafter. There was no protection if interferon was provided to the cells after infection. Treatment of the cells with interferon reduced the quantity of infectious progeny produced by the cells, reduced the number of cells producing infectious virus, and extended the length of the latent period. All infected cells, however, showed cytopathic changes.

Although the synthesis of herpes simplex virus in cell cultures can be in-hibited by interferon, it failed clinically to prevent or cure the replication of virus in the eyes of rabbits (CANTELL and TOMMILA, 1960).

XII. Essential Clinical Features
A. Herpes Simplex Virus

The diseases caused by this virus may be separated into two major types: (1) Pri-mary infections that occur in individuals who do not possess neutralizing anti-body in their bloodstream. (2) Recurrent infections that occur in individuals previously exposed to the virus and who possess antibodies against it.

Primary infections are usually systemic; in most cases, the infection is sub-clinical but it can be very severe and may be fatal. Viremia has been demonstrated in severe cases of primary herpetic infection (RUCHMAN and DODD, 1950).

Epidemiologic studies indicate that overt disease occurs in only about 10% to 15% of individuals with primary infections (SCOTT, 1957). The initial infection then subsides and the individual becomes a carrier with the virus in a latent state; recurrent disease may occur in such individuals as a result of a variety of nonspecific stimuli, such as fever, menstruation, ultraviolet light irradiation, gastro-intestinal upsets, and even psychic upsets. Patients with recurrent attack generally do not exhibit systemic symptoms and infection is localized.

1. Primary Herpes Simplex

The clinical expression of a primary infection is to a large degree dependent upon the portal of entry of the virus. The commonest form of clinical primary infection is acute herpetic *gingivostomatitis*, also called acute infectious gingivo-stomatitis, ulcerative stomatitis, and VINCENT's stomatitis. It occurs chiefly in children one to three years of age; it can also occur in older children and adults but never in younger children. The mucous membranes of the mouth are most frequently involved and the disease is characterized by fever, anorexia, and a sore mouth. The patients gums swell and redden and frequently bleed. There are lesions of the mucous membranes of the oral pharynx that appear first as white spots and then as ulcers; the breath becomes malodorous (DODD et al., 1938; SCOTT et al., 1941; ROGERS et al., 1949). The disease varies considerably in severity and length, is self-limiting, and disappears within about one to two weeks.

Another manifestation of primary herpes simplex infection is acute herpetic *vulvovaginitis*, in which lesions appear on the mucous membranes of the labia and lower vagina. The illness is accompanied by fever, local pain and inguinal adenopathy. The disease recedes in about one to two weeks (SLAVIN and GAVETT, 1946a). A counterpart to this disease in the male is *herpes progenitalis* in which grouped vesicles occur on the glans and the shaft of the penis.

Eczema herpeticum, also known as KAPOSI's varicelliform eruption, is a complication of eczema or atopic dermatitis in children; it is a serious disease and is frequently fatal. The illness starts abruptly with high fever and restlessness which is accompanied by the development of skin eruptions. Vesicles may appear and will remain for as long as a week or ten days. Death may occur from dehydration, secondary bacterial infection, or shock (BRAIN et al., 1957).

Infection of the eye with herpes simplex virus, *herpetic kerato-conjunctivitis* and *keratitis*, is a potentially serious disease that may lead to the loss of vision. The conjunctiva is inflamed and edematous while the cornea acquires a hazy appearance with superficial ulcerations. The eyelids are frequently closed and a purulent and membrane-like exudate appears. In the case of superficial involvement of the cornea, typical dendritic ulcers may develop and may result in sight impairment. The deep forms of the disease in the eye, disciform keratitis, hypopyon keratitis, and iridocyclitis may result in stromal lesions, as well as rupture of the cornea, and ends in serious scarring of the eye. The disease usually runs its course in about two to three weeks and may leave no residual damage to the cornea (THYGESON, 1959). Primary keratitis is more severe than the recurrent form of the disease.

Although herpes simplex virus can cause *meningo-encephalitis*, involvement of the central nervous system in infections with the virus is not common. The disease caused by this virus ranges from a mild aseptic meningitis to fatal encephalitis in which death occurs within one to two weeks. The disease begins with fever, headache, somnolence, stupor, and then convulsions, and in the case of encephalitis, delirium and coma. The cerebro-spinal fluid usually shows an increase in lymphocytes and there may be increased pressure. Herpes simplex virus has been implicated in about 10% of the cases of encephalitis (ADAIR et al., 1953; RAWLS et al., 1966; MILLER et al., 1966; LEIDER et al., 1965; KENT and NICHOLSON, 1964).

Primary infection also may sometimes occur by direct contact of herpes simplex virus with traumatic breaks (abrasions or lacerations) in normal skin, a frequent source of infection being the blisters on parents' lips. Vesicles generally appear at the site of the break and regional lymph adenopathy occurs. Fever may occur and usually subsides in a few days.

Generalized infection is a dangerous and usually fatal disease that occurs in premature and newborn infants (FLORMAN and MINDLIN, 1952; ZUELZER

and STULBERG, 1952; COLEBATCH, 1955; MACCALLUM, 1959). Infection of a
newborn may occur by transplacental infection during a primary infection of
the mother (MITCHELL and McCALL, 1963), as well as by passage through the
birth canal of a mother with primary herpetic vulvo-vaginitis (WHEELER and
HUFFINES, 1965). The infants develop a viremia that results in lesions in many
organs of the body, particularly in the viscera; this is associated with either
fever or hypothermia. Anorexia, vomiting, jaundice, lethargy, respiratory distress,
cyanosis and circulatory collapse then follow. The disease appears to be generally
fatal.

2. Recurrent Herpes Simplex

Recurrent herpes simplex of the skin, best known as cold sores or fever
blisters, as well as herpes labialis or febrilis, is characterized by eruptions of
groups of small, thin-walled, clear vesicles on an erythematous base, with local
itching or burning as the vesicles develop. These vesicles dry and form superficial crusts. The eruptions may occur on any part of the skin but occur most
frequently on the face, especially at muco-cutaneous junctions; they may also
occur on the penis (BARILE et al., 1962), in the urethra (ESTEVES and PINTO,
1952), on the vulva, buttocks, and thigh. Eruptions generally tend to recur in
the same places.

Kerato-conjunctivitis and traumatic herpes which first appear as primary
infections can also occur in recurrent form.

B. Pseudorabies Virus

The type of clinical manifestations observed in swine infected with pseudorabies
virus is dependent upon the age of the animals: in adult swine, there is generally
a mild, frequently subclinical, infection; in piglets (up until about 4 weeks of
age), the disease is severe and usually fatal.

In nature, pseudorabies is a highly contagious disease in swine. Although
in all other animals studied, there are usually signs of pruritis and nervous
involvement, most adult pigs undergo a mild febrile illness and do not exhibit
these signs. The incubation period varies from about three to eleven days. If there is
any nervous involvement (5% to 10% of the cases), the animals have a high fever,
are somnolent, and tend to vomit; the pigs develop a weakness and seem to
be close to death but usually recover within a week. The severe form of pseudorabies virus infection seems to be more prevalent in Europe than in the United
States. Weanling pigs react in about the same way as adults (AKKERMANS,
1963; SHOPE, 1964; McFERRAN and DOW, 1964a).

In piglets, the onset is sudden and entire litters may become ill and succumb
within 48 hours. The piglets may be affected while still *in utero*. GORDON and
LUKE (1955) infected a sow experimentally during the 10th week of pregnancy. The
sow gave birth to mummified fetuses 6 weeks later. Naturally infected sows
have also been shown to give birth to still-born animals (TERPSTRA, 1958). When
the animals are near 4 weeks of age, they show involvement of the nervous system
as indicated by an incoordination affecting the hindquarters that causes them
to move sideways. The disease of the central nervous system progresses rapidly,
ending in complete paralysis. There may also be spasmodic twitching of the

muscles and convulsive fits. The affected animals may exhibit respiratory distress, probably because of infection of the respiratory centers of the brain. The temperature is usually elevated (GORDON and LUKE, 1955).

Cattle infected with pseudorabies virus invariably die. The outstanding clinical feature in these animals is a severe pruritis with licking and rubbing of the affected sites (generally flanks, udders, and hindlegs) as a response to the irritation. As the central nervous system becomes involved, there is pharyngeal paralysis, increased salivation, and rapid labored respiration. Milk cows show a decrease in the output of milk. Many of the animals grind their teeth, bellow, become frenzied and aggressive, circle, and have a staggering gait, as well as partial paralysis of the hindquarters. The animals generally die within 48 hours after the first signs of disease appear (SHOPE, 1931; GALLOWAY, 1938; SHAHAN et al., 1947; Dow and McFERRAN, 1962a).

Other animals that are found infected naturally are sheep, dogs and cats. In general these animals show pruritis, involvement of the central nervous system; death occurs within a short time after the appearance of the first signs of the disease. Rabbits, mice and guinea pigs infected experimentally develop the same signs.

XIII. Pathology
A. Herpes Simplex Virus

The histological appearance of the lesions present in the tissues of patients with primary or recurrent infections is indistinguishable. The specific cellular changes are the same in all infected tissues and have been described in detail in the section on Cytopathology. In addition to the cytological alterations common to all tissues, cytopathic changes will occur that are characteristic for certain tissues. Thus, in the skin, the mucous membrane, the cornea, and the chorio-allantois of the chick embryo, there is a proliferation of the infected epithelial cells which thicken, become edematous, and eventually slough away, leaving an acute inflammatory, nonspecific ulceration. The changes in the skin are characterized by vesicle formation in the malpighian layer cells (SCOTT et al., 1950; SCOTT and TOKUMARU, 1965). The vesicles are filled with exudate containing infected epithelial cells, white blood cells, and necrotic cell debris. An inflammatory reaction occurs in the corium, with dilated blood vessels and cellular exudate. The mucosal lesion is similar. In generalized infections, the viscera are affected, including the liver and adrenals which show coagulation necrosis with cells surrounding the area presenting characteristic intranuclear inclusions. In the brain, the specific cytopathic changes cause the ultimate death of the infected cells, developing into areas of disintegrated neurons, as well as centers of necrosis with a surrounding inflammatory reaction.

B. Pseudorabies Virus

In swine, after intracerebral inoculation meningeal, perivascular and tissue infiltration are marked. There is also marked edema, variable amounts of diffuse cellular infiltration and microglial proliferation in the cerebral cortex; perivascular infiltration is markeded or necrotic neurons are present in the cortical areas. Intranuclear inclusions are found in the degenerating neurons and astrocytes (HURST, 1933; SHAHAN et al., 1947; Dow and McFERRAN, 1962b;

OLANDER et al., 1966). In naturally, as well as experimentally, infected swine, organs and tissues outside of the central nervous system show signs of infection; focal areas of necrosis have been found in liver, spleen, tonsils, epithelium of the tongue, soft palate, and other areas of the nasopharynx (GORDON and LUKE, 1955; CORNER, 1965; CSONTOS and SZÉKY, 1966).

In the rabbit, subcutaneous, intradermal, or intramuscular injection of virus leads to local inflammation and necrosis. The virus ascends the peripheral nerves to the corresponding ganglia and segments of the spinal cord, where primary degeneration of nerve and glial cells takes place. It is the destruction of the neurons that is probably responsible for the chief sign of the disease, pruritis. Death occurs soon after the virus reaches the medulla and before visible changes have been produced there. Intracerebral inoculation causes formation of characteristic lesions in the meninges, in subpial glial cells, and in superficially placed nerve cells. Intranuclear inclusions appear in all the cells.

The disease in guinea pigs follows the same course at that in rabbits. In monkeys there is widespread degeneration and necrosis of cortical nerve cells and the appearance of specific nuclear inclusions in nerve and glial cells after intra-cerebral inoculation. No lesions are found in the viscera. In the natural disease of cattle, the lesions are similar to those that appear in monkeys rather than to those of rabbits (HURST, 1933).

XIV. Diagnosis

A. Herpes Simplex Virus

1. Clinical Diagnosis

There are several diseases caused by viruses that produce vesicular eruptions on the skin, on the mucous membranes, or on both that may be confused with herpes simplex virus infections. The eczema caused by vaccinia may be distinguished from that caused by herpes simplex virus by the type of vesicles induced, as well as by the absence of intranuclear inclusions in the cells present in these vesicles. Varicella infection is best differentiated from herpes infection by virus isolation.

Although acute herpetic gingivostomatitis has a characteristic clinical appearance, it may be confused with herpangina caused by Coxsackie A virus. However, the distribution of the lesions differ — there is no gingivitis in Coxsackie infections, a typical feature of the herpes disease.

Herpes simplex virus-induced kerato-conjunctivitis may be distinguished from epidemic kerato-conjunctivitis caused by adenovirus chiefly by the fact that pain is a characteristic of the latter disease. Furthermore, if there is a history of recurrences, the disease may definitely be ascribed to herpes simplex virus.

It is practically impossible to differentiate meningoencephalitis caused by herpes from that caused by other viruses. These diseases can be distinguished only on the basis of laboratory diagnosis and, in fact, this is the best method for determining the cause of all these viral diseases.

2. Laboratory Diagnosis

There are a number of procedures that may be used to prove that herpes simplex virus is the agent responsible for one of the diseases described above.

Infectious virus may be isolated from lesions, blood, or various tissues of the body at autopsy and identified as herpes simplex virus by inoculation into susceptible animals, such as embryonated eggs, mice (especially the newborn), rabbits, guinea pigs, hamsters, cotton rats, and day-old chicks, which develop infections characteristic for this virus. The virus may also be grown in primary rabbit kidney and chick embryo cell cultures, as well as in HeLa cells and primary human amnion cells. These cells will show cytopathic changes characteristic for herpes simplex virus. Identification of the virus may also be made by the direct visualization of viral particles after staining with phosphotungstic acid in the electron microscope (SMITH and MELNICK, 1962). Viral antigen in infected cells taken from vesicles or the cornea may be identified with specific fluorescent antiserum (BIEGELEISEN et al., 1959; KAUFMAN, 1960).

In the case of primary infections, in which there is an increase in specific antibody against the virus, sera of individuals suspected of having a herpetic infection may be tested for a rise in neutralizing antibody (TOKUMARU and SCOTT, 1964) and in complement fixing antibody (HAYWARD, 1950; Ross et al., 1964). In addition to the usual neutralizing antibody that appears after a primary infection, it has been found recently that a neutralizing antibody appears in rabbits that can be detected only in the presence of complement (YOSHINO and TANIGUCHI, 1964 and 1965; TANIGUCHI and YOSHINO, 1965). Detection of this complement-requiring neutralizing antibody may be used as a means for the early diagnosis of herpetic infections (YOSHINO and TANIGUCHI, 1966).

Confirmation of suspected cases of herpes infection may also be made by means of a skin test in which an erythema and induration of 5 mm or greater in diameter develops in the skin (NAGLER, 1944; JAWETZ et al., 1951; ANDERSON and KILBOURNE, 1961 b). This test is reliable for individuals between the ages of 5 and 50 (SCOTT, 1957).

B. Pseudorabies Virus

1. Clinical Diagnosis

The disease in cattle is so characteristic (see above) that laboratory confirmation is usually not necessary. Clinical diagnosis is, however, much more difficult in adult swine infected with pseudorabies virus, especially since the overt disease is not common in these animals. Suckling pigs or young swine, which succumb in a coma or with signs of involvement of the central nervous system, should be suspected of being infected with pseudorabies virus.

2. Laboratory Diagnosis

Classically, diagnosis of pseudorabies virus infections in animals has been made by inoculation of infected material into rabbits which undergo a characteristic disease and die. Rats (SHOPE, 1935) and chick embryos (BANG, 1942) may also be used for this purpose. Virus can also be isolated in cultures of chick embryo cells (BÉLÁDI and SZÖLLŐSY, 1955) and rabbit kidney cells (KAPLAN and VATTER, 1959). Virus can be isolated in cell culture from a variety of organs of infected animals, including tonsils, brain, lungs, and a number of others (MASIČ et al., 1965; CSONTOS, 1966; PETTE, 1965; ŠKODA and ŽUFFA, 1962).

Evidence that an animal has had an infection with pseudorabies virus may be provided by testing the serum of the animal for the presence of neutralizing (KAPLAN and VATTER, 1959) and complement-fixing antibodies (NACHKOV et al., 1958) in the same manner as done for herpes simplex virus.

XV. Treatment

Nonspecific, systemic supportive therapy may be required in some cases of primary infection with herpes simplex virus to prevent the possibility of death. These measures consist generally of transfusion of parenteral fluids, plasma and blood transfusions, plus symptomatic measures and good nursing care. In some cases, γ-globulin as a prophylactic measure for infants with eczema has been suggested (SCOTT and TOKUMARU, 1965). The prevention of acidosis and dehydration in infants with severe gingivostomatitis and especially with eczema is extremely important.

Successful chemotherapy of herpes keratitis in man and rabbits by IUdR and Ara-C has been reported (KAUFMAN, 1962; KAUFMAN et al. 1962; UNDERWOOD, 1962; UNDERWOOD et al., 1964). Most subsequent studies confirmed these initial results and a number of double-blind studies, carefully carried out, showed that IUdR had a significant effect on superficial herpes keratitis but that it failed to heal all superficial lesions, to reduce significantly the recurrence rate, or to prevent the development of stromal lesions (BURNS, 1963; PATTERSON et al., 1963; LEOPOLD, 1963; LAIBSON and LEOPOLD, 1964; JEPSON, 1964; PAYROU and DOHLMAN, 1964; POLACK and ROSE, 1964; HART et al., 1965). However, there were some studies that indicated that there was no significant difference between the controls and those treated with IUdR (LUNTZ and MacCALLUM, 1963).

Prolonged therapy with IUdR may lead to the selection of mutants of herpes simplex virus resistant to the action of the drug (UNDERWOOD et al., 1964; KOBAYASHI and NAKAMURA, 1964); however, these virus mutants are still sensitive to the action of Ara-C, a drug, which although effective in the control of herpes keratitis, seems to be slower than IUdR in clearing the initial infection and is considerably more toxic than IUdR to the host cells (KAUFMAN et al., 1964; KAUFMAN, 1965; UNDERWOOD et al., 1965). IUdR has also been tested for its capacity to cure cutaneous infections caused by herpes simplex virus. Although one controlled, double-blind study failed to demonstrate any therapeutic effect of the drug (BURNETT and KATZ, 1963), a study with rabbits, in whose skin fever blister-like lesions were produced, indicated that IUdR did show some promise in preventing lesion formation (FORCE et al., 1964). Treatment with IUdR appeared also to ameliorate herpes progenitalis (SCHOFIELD, 1964).

XVI. Epidemiology
A. Herpes Simplex Virus

In 1930, ANDREWES and CARMICHAEL observed that about three-fourths of a group of 53 normal adults possessed neutralizing antibody to herpes simplex virus and that 7 patients with frequently recurring herpes labialis all had antibody in their sera. Later studies by DODD et al. (1938) and BURNET and WILLIAMS

(1939) showed that children without neutralizing antibody developed stomatitis as a result of infection with herpes simplex virus; on recovery these children developed antibodies against the virus. Thus, it was soon realized that the population is divided into two groups with respect to the natural diseases caused by herpes simplex virus: (1) One group does not possess antibody against the virus and is susceptible to primary infection; (2) a second group does possess antibody and is subject to recurrent infection.

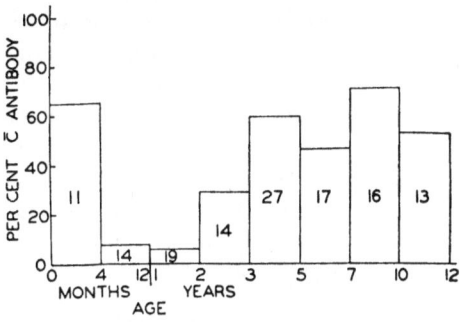

1. Primary Infection

a) Age Distribution

A correlation exists between the level of neutralizing and complement-fixing antibodies in individuals and their susceptibility to infection with

Fig. 13. Distribution of neutralizing antibodies to herpes simplex virus in a population of 121 children. The number in each bar indicates the number of children tested at each age group. From T. F. McNair Scott et al., J. Pediat. **41**, 835 (1952).

herpes simplex virus. In contrast to the general population of which 60% to 100% possess antibodies, few children do (WEYER, 1932; BURNET and LUSH, 1939a; SCOTT et al., 1952; BUDDINGH et al., 1953; TATENO et al., 1958; HAYWARD, 1950; HOLZEL et al., 1953; DASCOMB et al., 1965; SCHMIDT and LENNETTE, 1961; BECKER, 1966; YOSHINO et al., 1962). As Fig. 13 shows, few children

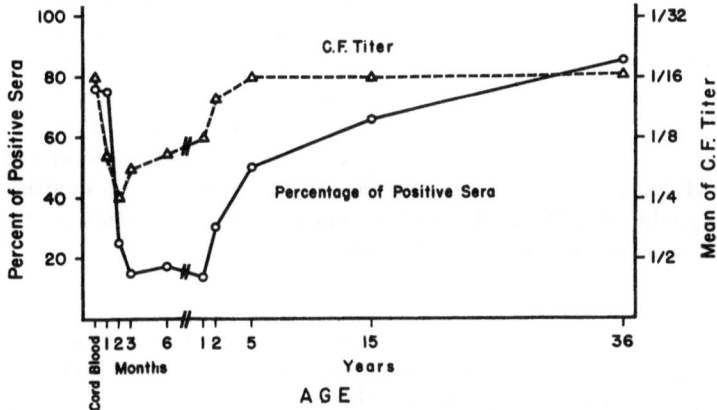

Fig. 14. Distribution of complement-fixing antibodies to herpes simplex virus at different ages, as determined from tests on 304 sera. Adapted from A. HOLZEL et al., Acta paediat. **42**, 206 (1953).

between the ages of 4 months and 2 years have neutralizing antibodies, which is also the period of the greatest susceptibility to primary infection with herpes virus. By the age of 5, more than half the population possesses neutralizing antibody. From the data in Fig. 13, it also appears that antibodies are transmitted via the placenta from immune mothers to their infants and persist in infants for about 5 to 6 months. Complement-fixing antibodies follow the same general trend as the neutralizing antibodies (Fig. 14). Between 6 months and the end of the first year, *eczema herpeticum* may occur; acute herpetic *gingivo-*

stomatitis is most prevalent between 1 and 3 years. Offspring of mothers without circulating antibody generally are susceptible to infection from birth and represent the group among which neo-natal herpes occurs most often.

The age distribution of herpes keratitis, a serious disease, which is now the most important eye disease leading to loss of vision in the United States (THY-GESON et al., 1953), is somewhat different from the other infections caused by herpes simplex virus. Two-thirds of the cases of herpetic keratitis occurs between the ages of 40 and 70, the highest incidence being in the 41 to 60 year age group. Males appear to predominate in this age bracket but there appears to be an equal distribution between the sexes in the earlier decades (GOLD et al., 1965). The rate of recurrence of this disease is about 25% and patients, who had more than one attack, have a good probability (43%) of an additional recurrence within 2 years (CARROLL et al., 1967).

b) Socio-economic Distribution

In their serological survey, ANDREWES and CARMICHAEL (1930) found that the number of medical students possessing neutralizing antibodies to herpes simplex virus was lower than that in the general population of a hospital. This difference in the proportion of positive sera in different socio-economic classes was pursued by BURNET and LUSH (1939a) who reported that 51 out of 55 (93%) of patients at a public hospital compared to 16 out of 37 (43%) of graduates and students at this hospital had neutralizing antibodies.

An extensive analysis of the effect of socio-economic factors on the epidemiology of herpes simplex virus infection was carried out in South Africa by BECKER (1966) who examined the distribution of neutralizing antibodies among three racial groups, white, colored and Bantu. His results were consistent with the notion that there is an inverse relationship between socio-economic status and the rate of acquisition of neutralizing antibodies by the population, a reflection of poor hygiene and overcrowding. There was also a striking association between primary disseminated herpes simplex virus infection in children (6 to 25 months of age) and severe grades of malnutrition or kwashiorkor, clearly conditions found only in the lower socio-economic levels (BECKER et al., 1963).

c) Reservoir of Virus

The reservoir of herpes simplex virus is man himself. Most infections with this virus appear to be subclinical; it has been estimated by SCOTT (1957) that at least 90% of the infections fall into this category. The subclinical nature of the disease is emphasized by the fact that it is rare to find a case of infection to have been caused by a known contact (SCOTT, 1957). It is evident, therefore, that the reservoir of infection consists of individuals who have either had the disease and have recovered but continue to shed virus, or of individuals who shed virus without ever having had overt disease.

Virus has been isolated from children who have had herpes stomatitis 23 weeks post infection, a time when there was no clinical evidence of disease (SCOTT and STEIGMAN, 1941). The saliva and stools of children, who have fully recovered from infection, have also been found to contain virus up to 23 days, on the average, after infection. Furthermore, the saliva of individuals, who have no clinical manifestations of disease, may also contain the virus. The presence of virus in the saliva decreases with increasing age: of 571 individuals tested, 20% of the children 7 months to 2 years of age, but only 2.5% of the group 15 years of age or over had virus in their saliva (BUDDINGH et al., 1953).

d) Incubation Period

The incubation period ranges from about two to twelve days with a mean of 6.2 ± 2.7 days (JURETIC, 1960; HALE et al., 1963).

e) Epidemics

Epidemics of disease caused by herpes simplex virus are not common, since, as indicated above, more than 90% of the infections due to this virus are sub-clinical and the major part of the population has antibodies against the virus. Nevertheless, there have been a few reports of epidemics of primary herpetic infections. SCOTT and STEIGMAN (1941) described an epidemic that occurred within 3 families, and PUGH et al. (1955) one that occurred in the ward of a hospital. ANDERSON and HAMILTON (1949) found an attack rate of 56% in an orphanage in Australia, and HALE et al. (1963) an attack rate of 77% in an orphanage in the United States.

f) Transmission of Infection

The spread of herpes simplex virus infections appears to occur primarily by direct contact, most likely by way of the saliva or oral secretions (BUDDINGH et al., 1953). Adults with vesicles about their lips may transmit the infection by kissing children, because the skin and mucous membranes of children are probably highly susceptible to infection with herpes simplex virus (BURNET, 1945). Primary infection may develop in children who have come in contact with the virus after traumatic breaks in their skin caused by burns or abrasions. Primary infections in the adult may also occur by kissing or by sexual intercourse (SLAVIN and GAVETT, 1946a).

2. Recurrent Infections

Individuals who suffer from recurrent infections with herpes simplex virus have antibodies against this agent. The titer of antibody in these persons does not appear to change despite repeated recurrent attacks. One of the more interesting aspects of the epidemiology of recurrent herpes infections is the fact that this virus tends to go into a latent state in individuals recovering from primary infection. Recurrent infections occur only after induction by some internal or external environmental factor. The nature of the latent state of herpes simplex virus will be discussed in detail below.

B. Pseudorabies Virus

There have been many outbreaks of infection in domestic animals caused by pseudorabies virus that have reached epidemic proportions. These epidemics have been world wide in distribution, and no continent has been left untouched (BURGGRAAF and LOURENS, 1932; SHOPE, 1935a and b; GALLOWAY, 1938; RAY, 1943; LAMONT, 1946; GORDON and LUKE, 1955; SHAHAN et al., 1947; TONEVA,

1958; Saunders and Gustafson, 1964; Janowski and Oberfeld, 1965; Škoda and Grunert, 1965; Akkermans, 1963). The epidemics are characterized, in general, by the development of a mild, febrile disease in adult swine and fatal infections in suckling pigs, cattle and sheep. There is, however, some mortality among growing and mature swine, a condition which has been prevalent in Europe and which recently has been increasing in the United States (Saunders et al., 1963; Gustafson and Saunders, 1966).

Pseudorabies virus causes a highly contagious disease in swine; the incubation period of this disease varies from about 3 to 11 days in these animals. The virus probably spreads from pig to pig via nasal discharges; virus can be demonstrated in the nose of swine for periods of time varying between 2 and 17 days (McFerran and Dow, 1964a; Csontos, 1964; Shope, 1964). Sows are often responsible for spreading the disease to their offspring (Kojnok, 1965), possibly via the mother's milk (Kojnok, 1957). The virus may also be transmitted between male and female swine during coitus (Akkermans, 1963).

Neutralizing antibodies against pseudorabies virus develop in swine that recover from infection. Although Shope (1964) has suggested that most herds of adult swine in Midwestern United States possess neutralizing antibodies, indicating that the animals are resistant to infection, Saunders and Gustafson (1964) have found recently that most of the swine population of Indiana does not possess neutralizing antibody. They found that of the serum samples taken from 271 swine (representing 104 herds from 54 counties), only 4 (representing 2 herds from 2 counties) were positive.

In the herds of swine that possess neutralizing antibody, there is transfer of maternal antibody to newborn pigs by way of the colostrum, as well as by way of the mother's milk and the antibodies persist in the piglets for about 5 to 7 weeks (Kojnok and Surjan, 1963). This provides protection to the piglets during the most susceptible period of their existence, probably reducing infection to the subclinical state. However, piglets born of non-immune mothers are susceptible and may contract the overt form of the disease. Thus, when the disease does occur in neonatal pigs, one may consider the outbreak to be the result of an introduction of virus into a susceptible herd of swine at approximately the time that the pigs are undergoing parturition. The older swine in the herd will also be infected but will show a subclinical form of the disease.

Swine probably constitute the natural reservoir of pseudorabies virus. There are many data in the literature indicating that virus spreads directly from pigs to cattle and sheep (see Kojnok, 1962). A recent, careful investigation by Kojnok (1962) seems quite definitely to establish this point. The sheep and cattle that came down with the disease had been housed in the same quarters with swine that had exhibited signs of pseudorabies virus infection. Most of the swine had neutralizing antibodies against pseudorabies virus; none of the surviving cattle or sheep did. It is quite evident that one prophylactic measure that may be taken against disease is to house pigs separately from the other animals on the farm.

How the virus spreads from farm to farm is not known precisely. It has been assumed that rats may play a role in the spread of the virus because virus has been isolated from these animals (Shope, 1935a). Cases of pseudorabies virus infection in rat-terrier dogs which were believed to have killed rats on a pig farm in Ireland have been reported (LAMONT and GORDON, 1950). The dogs may have carried the disease to other farms.

XVII. Latent and Persistent Virus

Perhaps one of the most interesting features of the herpes simplex and pseudo-rabies viruses is that following the initial infection, the virus disappears and enters into a quiescent, latent state. Infection recurs only as a reaction to certain stimuli. External factors such as irradiation or skin irradiation, as well as internal factors, such as certain pyrogenic-inducing diseases, will cause the development of facial herpes. The disease has also been produced by artificially induced fever (CARPENTER et al., 1940). Menstruation (SCOTT, 1957), injury to nerves (CARTON and KILBOURNE, 1952), as well as emotional factors (BLANK and BRODY, 1950; SCHNECK, 1947), also play a role in the recurrence of the disease. Sometimes treatment of patients with anti-inflammatory steroids may induce the recurrence of corneal infections from healed herpetic keratitis (LEOPOLD and SERY, 1963).

These epidemiological and clinical observations on the propensity of the viruses of the herpes group to enter into a quiescent state from which they can be induced to appear in an active form have been complemented by experimental observations of rabbits infected with herpes simplex virus. In one set of experiments, rabbits were sensitized with egg white and were later inoculated with virus intramuscularly. Animals that recovered from the infection were shocked anaphylactically one to three months after infection. This treatment reactivated the latent herpetic infections and virus could be recovered from the central nervous system of the animals (GOOD and CAMPBELL, 1945 and 1948). Reactivation of latent herpes simplex virus encephalitis in rabbits was also obtained by inoculating the animals with adrenalin (SCHMIDT and RASMUSSEN, 1960b).

Reactivation of herpes simplex virus in healed rabbit corneal lesions was induced experimentally (ANDERSON et al., 1961). In these experiments, the animals were sensitized to horse serum and an Arthus reaction was induced in the healed corneas. In seven out of nineteen attempts at induction, virus was repeatedly recovered from swabbings taken from the corneas, although herpes keratitis was not observed. The reactivation of herpes keratitis in healed corneas has been accomplished by inoculating the animals with epinephrine at a distant site (LAIBSON and KIBRICK, 1966).

Although virus can generally be isolated after the induction of localized cell necrosis, it has not been isolated from recurrently infected areas during periods between infections (FINDLAY and MacCALLUM, 1940; ANDERSON and HAMILTON, 1949; RUSTIGIAN et al., 1966). However, virus has been isolated from the tears and saliva of normal human beings, as well as from the secretory glands and tears of rabbits, who suffered from recurrent herpes keratitis, despite the normal appearance of the eyes. These observations have led to the notion that perhaps recurrent herpes infections are due to the chronic multiplication of the virus in such organs as the lachrymal and salivary glands, rather than to the reactivation of localized latent infection (KAUFMAN et al., 1967).

The persistence of virus, as well as the recurrence of the disease in individuals that possess antibodies against the virus, may be explained by the finding that herpes simplex virus can move from cell to cell directly without coming in contact with the extracellular milieu. However, the phenomenon of latency and reactivation still remains unexplained.

A number of hypotheses have been put forward to account for the latent infection of man with herpes simplex virus. PAINE (1964) proposed that after primary infection, the virus remains in a latent state in the sensory ganglia. On activation, the virus moves down the axon of the peripheral nerve to the epithelial cells. HERRIOTT (1961) has considered the possibility that cells may be infected by free infectious viral DNA. Infection could thus occur in the presence of specific anti-viral serum which affects intact virus only. The reason for the submergence of the virus between episodes could, according to HERRIOTT, be the presence of humoral nucleases. Under conditions of stress these nucleases would become inhibited; thus, the area of infection would be enlarged and symptoms would be produced. However, that free viral DNA plays a role in the infectivity of the virus is an unlikely possibility, since it has never been found outside the nucleus of infected cells. Furthermore, since the molecules of DNA of herpes virus are relatively large, the transmission from cell to cell of intact molecules would most likely be a rare occurrence.

The possibility that herpes simplex virus and pseudorabies virus may exist as proviruses within the host cell in the same manner as prophage does in lysogenic bacteria has been considered by many investigators and has stimulated the examination of the relationship of these viruses to susceptible cells cultivated *in vitro*. Both herpes simplex virus and pseudorabies virus were found to behave like "virulent" viruses and, in general, cells infected with these viruses do not survive. One notable exception, however, has been reported. HAMBURG and SVET-MOLDAVSKY (1964) infected Sarcoma-237 tumor cells with herpes simplex virus *in vitro* and showed that the tumor cells did not grow when implanted in mice that had been pre-immunized against herpes simplex virus, although the tumor cells did grow in control mice vaccinated against vaccinia virus or in nonimmunized animals. These results imply that the cells survived infection with herpes simplex virus and became "transformed", so that they reacted with antiserum against viral antigen.

Although the evidence that the viruses of the herpes group may exist in a provirus state has, in general, been negative, the investigation of this problem has led to a number of interesting observations on the persistence of herpes simplex virus in cultures of susceptible cells cultivated *in vitro*.

Persistently infected cultures can be obtained by inoculating them at low virus: cell ratios, and by the addition of virus-specific antiserum to the medium. As long as the antiserum is present, the cultures survive and the infection is maintained at a low level by cell to cell transfer of infectious material. When the antiserum is removed from the cultures, infection becomes rampant throughout the cultures and most of the cells are destroyed. Some cells, however, survive, and these are more resistant to reinfection with the virus. Persistent infections of this type have been reported for a variety of herpes simplex virus-cell systems (WHEELER, 1960; FERNANDEZ, 1960; HINZE and WALKER, 1961a; SZÁNTÓ, 1963).

It has also been found that cultures could be persistently infected with herpes simplex virus in the absence of antiserum. The conditions essential for the maintenance of a balanced state between the proliferation of the cells and of the virus were a low level of cellular metabolic activity and a very small virus inoculum (COLEMAN and JAWETZ, 1961; GÉDER et al., 1965). Similar results were obtained by BÉLÁDI and BAKAY (1963) and by SOMOGYIOVÁ (1965) for pseudorabies virus-infected calf kidney cells. Persistently infected cultures could be maintained in the presence of calf serum, although no virus neutralizing antibodies were present in this serum. The fact that a small virus inoculum is essential for the establishment of a persistently infected culture indicates that interferon may play a role in this phenomenon.

One interesting type of persistent infection was obtained with the herpes simplex virus infected-Chinese hamster cell system. These cultures were persistently infected *in vitro* with cycles of cell lysis and cell growth in the absence of virus-specific antiserum. Regrowth and destruction of cells by herpes simplex virus occurred simultaneously in the same cultures but in different areas. This was most likely due to the selection of resistant cells which then divided and gave rise to mixed populations of resistant, as well as susceptible, cells (HAMPAR and COPELAND, 1965; HAMPAR, 1966a and b).

Although the experiments just described may provide models of "latent" infection, their exact bearing on recurring herpes simplex virus infection in man is not clear, and the elucidation of the phenomenon of latent infection with this virus still requires a great deal of study.

XVIII. Abbreviations

Ara-C, 1-β-D-arabinofuranosylcytosine; BUdR, 5-bromo-2′-deoxyuridine; CUdR, 5-chloro-2′-deoxyuridine; DNase, deoxyribonuclease; HEp-2, human epidermoid carcinoma No. 2; IUdR, 5-iodo-2′-deoxyuridine; PFU, plaque-forming unit; RNase, ribonuclease; TMP, thymidine monophosphate.

References

ADAIR, C. V., R. L. GAULD, and J. E. SMADEL: Aseptic meningitis, a disease of diverse etiology: clinical and etiologic studies on 854 cases. Ann. intern. Med. **39**, 675—704 (1953).

AKKERMANS, J. P. W. M.: Ziekte van Aujeszky bit het varken in Nederland. Monograph (1963).

ALBRECHT, P., J. BLAŠKOVIČ, J. JAKUBIK, and J. LEŠŠO: Demonstration of pseudorabies virus in chick embryo cell cultures and infected animals by the fluorescent antibody technique. Acta virol. **7**, 289—296 (1963).

ALLEN, E. G., B. KANEDA, A. J. GIRARDI, T. F. McN. SCOTT, and M. M. SIGEL: Preservation of viruses of the psittacosis-lymphogranuloma venerum group and herpes simplex under various conditions of storage. J. Bact. **63**, 369—376 (1952).

AMOS, H.: The inactivation of herpes simplex virus by phosphatase enzymes. J. exp. Med. 98, 365—372 (1953).

ANDERSON, K.: Pathogenesis of herpes simplex virus infection in chick embryos. Amer. J. Path. **16**, 137—155 (1940).

ANDERSON, K.: Dual virus infection of single cells. Amer. J. Path. **18**, 577—583 (1942).

ANDERSON, S. G., and J. HAMILTON: The epidemiology of primary herpes simplex infection. Med. J. Aust. **36**, 308—311 (1949).

ANDERSON, S. G., J. HAMILTON, and S. WILLIAMS: An attempt to vaccinate against herpes simplex. Aust. J. exp. Biol. med. Sci. **28**, 579—584 (1950).

ANDERSON, W. A., and E. D. KILBOURNE: Immunization of mice with inactivated herpes simplex virus. Proc. Soc. exp. Biol. (N.Y.) **107**, 518—520 (1961a).

ANDERSON, W. A., and E. D. KILBOURNE: A herpes simplex skin test diagnostic antigen of low protein content from cell culture fluid. J. invest. Derm. **37**, 25—28 (1961b).

ANDERSON, W. A., B. MARGRUDER, and E. D. KILBOURNE: Induced reactivation of herpes simplex virus in healed rabbit corneal lesions. Proc. Soc. exp. Biol. (N.Y.) **107**, 628—632 (1961).

ANDERVONT, H. B.: Activity of herpetic virus in mice. J. infect. Dis. **44**, 383—393 (1929a).

ANDERVONT, H. B.: Pathogenicity of two strains of herpetic virus for mice. J. infect. Dis. **45**, 366—385 (1929b).

ANDREWES, C. H.: Tissue-culture in the study of immunity to herpes. J. Path. Bact. **33**, 302—312 (1930).

ANDREWES, C. H.: Classification of viruses of vertebrates. Advanc. Virus Res. **9**, 271—296 (1962).

ANDREWES, C. H., and M. B. CARMICHAEL: A note on the presence of antibodies to herpes virus in post-encephalitic and other human sera. Lancet **1**, 857—858 (1930).

ANDREWES, C. H., and D. M. HORSTMANN: The susceptibility of viruses to ethyl ether. J. gen. Microbiol. **3**, 290—297 (1949).

ANTONELLI, A., M. MAZZOTTI e I. ARCHETTI: Studio sulle condizioni di conservazione del virus erpetico. R. C. Ist. sup. Sanità **27**, 185—190 (1964).

ARMSTRONG, J. A., H. G. PEREIRA, and C. H. ANDREWES: Observations on the virus of infectious bovine rhinotracheitis, and its affinity with the *Herpesvirus* group. Virology **14**, 276—285 (1961).

ASHE, W. K., and H. W. SCHERP: Antigenic analysis of herpes simplex virus by neutralization kinetics. J. Immunol. **91**, 658—665 (1963).

ASHE, W. K., and H. W. SCHERP: Antigenic variations in herpes simplex virus isolates from successive recurrences of herpetic labialis. J. Immunol. **94**, 385—394 (1965).

AUJESZKY, A.: Über eine neue Infektionskrankheit bei Haustieren. Zbl. Bakt. I. Abt. Orig. **32**, 353—373 (1902).

AURELIAN, L., and B. ROIZMAN: The host range of herpes simplex virus: interferon, viral DNA, and antigen synthesis in abortive infection of dog kidney cells. Virology **22**, 452—461 (1964).

AURELIAN, L., and B. ROIZMAN: Abortive infection of canine cells by herpes simplex virus. II. Alternative suppression of synthesis of interferon and viral constituents. J. molec. Biol. **11**, 539—548 (1965).

AURELIAN, L., and R. R. WAGNER: Two populations of herpes virus virions which appear to differ in physical properties and DNA composition. Proc. nat. Acad. Sci. (Wash.) **56**, 902—909 (1966).

BAHR, O. F.: Electron stains. III. Osmium tetroxide and ruthenium tetroxide and their reactions with biologically important substances. Exp. Cell Res. **7**, 457—479 (1954).

BAILLY, J.: Maladie d'Aujeszky in "Les Ultravirus des Maladies Animales" (LEVADITI, LÉPINE et VERGE, eds.), pp. 703—727, Paris: Librairie Maloine, 1938.

BAKER, W. H., A. M. LAWTON, and K. MCCARTHY: Primary generalized infection caused by herpes simplex virus. Brit. med. J. **2**, 1334—1336 (1952).

BALDELLI, B., F. DE MAJO, T. FRESCRUA e P. CARDARAS: La pseudo-rabbia (malatti di Aujeszky) nei suini: accertamenti diagnostici e profilassi immunizzante. Nuovi Ann. Ig. **15**, 23—30 (1964).

BANG, F. B.: Experimental infection of the chick embryo with the virus of pseudorabies. J. exp. Med. **76**, 263—270 (1942).

BARILE, M. F., J. M. BLUMBERG, C. W. KRAUL, and R. YAGUCHI: Penile lesions among U.S. armed forces personnel in Japan. Arch. Derm. **86**, 273—281 (1962).

BARÓCSAI, G., and D. TANCZER: Experiences on active immunization against Aujeszky's disease. Magy. Állatorv. Lap. **17**, 350—351 (1962).

BARON, S., and H. B. LEVY: Interferon. Ann. Rev. Microbiol. **20**, 291—318 (1966).

BARSKI, G.: Interférence entre les virus d'herpès et de polyome chez le hamster adulte *in vivo*. C. R. Acad. Sci. (Paris) **256**, 5459—5462 (1963).

BARSKI, G., and FR. CORNEFERT: Response of different mouse cell strains to polyoma infection *in vitro*. Latency and self-inhibition effect in infected cultures. J. nat. Cancer Inst. **28**, 823—843 (1962).

BARSKI, G., M. LAMY et P. LÉPINE: Culture de cellules trypsinées de rein de lapin et leur application a l'étude des virus du group herpétique. Ann. Inst. Pasteur **89**, 415—427 (1955).

BARSKI, G., and R. ROBINEAUX: Evolution of herpes simplex cellular lesions observed *in vitro* by phase contrast microcinematography. Proc. Soc. exp. Biol. (N.Y.) **101**, 632—636 (1959).

BARTHA, A.: Experiments to reduce the virulence of Aujeszky's virus. Magy. Állatorv. Lap. **16**, 42—45 (1961).

BARTHA, A., and J. KOJNOK: Immunization experiments with the attenuated strain of Aujeszky's virus. Magy. Állatorv. Lap. (September), 321—323 (1962).

BAUMGARTNER, G.: Infektionsversuche mit isolierten oxychromatischen Einschlüssen des Herpes. Schweiz. med. Wschr. **16**, 759—760 (1935).

BECHHOLD, H., und M. SCHLESINGER: Die Größenbestimmung von Herpes-Virus durch Zentrifugierversuche. Z. Hyg. Infekt.-Kr. **115**, 342—353 (1933).

BECKER, W.: The epidemiology of herpesvirus infection in three racial communities in Cape Town. S. Afr. med. J. **40**, 109—111 (1966).

BECKER, W., T. DU NAUDÉ, A. KIPPS, and D. MCKENZIE: Virus studies in disseminated herpes simplex infections. Association with malnutrition in children. S. Afr. med. J. **37**, 74—76 (1963).

BEDSON, S. P.: Immunization with killed herpes virus. Brit. J. exp. Path. **12**, 254—260 (1931).

BEDSON, S. P., and G. J. CRAWFORD: Immunity in experimental herpes. Brit. J. exp. Path. **8**, 138—147 (1927).

BEDSON, S. P., and J. V. T. GOSTLING: Further observations on the mode of multiplication of herpes virus. Brit. J. exp. Path. **39**, 502—509 (1958).

BÉLÁDI, I.: Study on the plaque formation and some properties of the Aujeszky disease virus on chicken embryo cells. Acta vet. Acad. Sci. hung. **12**, 417—422 (1962).

BÉLÁDI, I., and M. BAKAY: Persistent pseudorabies virus infection in calf cells. Acta virol. **7**, 477 (1963).

BÉLÁDI, I., und G. IVÁNOVICS: Immunisierung von Laboratoriumstieren mit dem Virus der Aujeszky'schen Krankheit nach dessen Inaktivierung mit Ultraviolettstrahlen. Acta microbiol. Acad. Sci. hung. **11**, 151—160 (1954).

BÉLÁDI, I., and E. SZÖLLÖSY: Production in monolayer tissue culture by Aujeszky-disease (pseudorabies) virus. Acta microbiol. Acad. Sci. hung. **3**, 213—217 (1955).

BELTZ, R. E.: Comparison of the content of thymidylate synthetase, deoxycytidylate deaminase and deoxyribonucleoside kinases in normal and regenerating rat liver. Arch. Biochem. **99**, 304—312 (1962).

BENDA, R.: Attempt to differentiate B virus from herpes simplex virus by the fluorescent antibody technique. Acta virol. **10**, 348—353 (1966).

BEN-PORAT, T., and A. S. KAPLAN: The chemical composition of herpes simplex and pseudorabies viruses. Virology **16**, 261—266 (1962).

BEN-PORAT, T., and A. S. KAPLAN: The synthesis and fate of pseudorabies virus DNA in infected mammalian cells in the stationary phase of growth. Virology **20**, 310—317 (1963).

BEN-PORAT, T., and A. S. KAPLAN: Mechanism of inhibition of cellular DNA synthesis by pseudorabies virus. Virology **25**, 22—29 (1965).

BERRY, G. P., and H. B. SLAVIN: Studies on herpetic infection in mice. I. Passive protection against virus inoculated nasally. J. exp. Med. **78**, 305—312 (1943).

BESWICK, T. S. L.: Experimental herpes simplex infection in the baby mouse. J. Path. Bact. 76, 133—142 (1958).

BESWICK, T. S. L.: The origin and the use of the word herpes. Med. Hist. 6, 214—232 (1962).

BEVERIDGE, W. I. B., and F. M. BURNET: The cultivation of viruses and rickettsiae in the chick embryo. Spec. Rep. Ser. med. Res. Coun. (Lond.) No. 258 (1946).

BIEGELEISEN, J. Z., L. H. RILEY, JR., and L. V. SCOTT: Isolation of herpes simplex virus from the blood of rabbits. Virology 4, 182—183 (1957).

BIEGELEISEN, J. Z., JR., L. V. SCOTT, and V. LEWIS, JR.: Rapid diagnosis of herpes simplex virus infections with fluorescent antibody. Science 129, 640—641 (1959).

BLACK, F. L., and J. L. MELNICK: Micro-epidemiology of poliomyelitis and herpes-B infections — spread of the viruses within tissue cultures. J. Immunol. 74, 236—242 (1955).

BLANK, H., and M. W. BRODY: Recurrent herpes simplex, a psychiatric and laboratory study. Psychosom. Med. 12, 254—260 (1950).

BLANK, H., C. F. BURGOON, G. D. BALDRIDGE, P. L. McCARTHY, and F. URBACH: Cytologic smears in diagnosis of herpes simplex, herpes zoster, and varicella. J. Amer. med. Ass. 146, 1410—1412 (1951).

BOIRON, M., J. TANZER, M. THOMAS, and A. HAMPE: Early diffuse chromosome alterations in monkey kidney cells infected in vitro with herpes simplex virus. Nature (Lond.) 209, 737—738 (1966).

BOJARSKI, T. B., and H. H. HIATT: Stabilization of thymidylate kinase activity by thymidylate and thymidine. Nature (Lond.) 188, 1112—1114 (1960).

BONET-MAURY, P.: Irradiation et méthodes statistiques de titrage des ultravirus. In "Les Ultravirus des Maladies Animales" (LEVADITI, LÉPINE et VERGE, eds.), p. 165. Paris: S. A. Maloine (Libraire). 1948.

BOSCH, L., E. HARBERS, and C. HEIDELBERGER: Studies on fluorinated pyrimidines. V. Effects on nucleic acid metabolism in vitro. Cancer Res. 18, 335—343 (1958).

BRAIN, R. T.: Biological therapy in virus diseases. Brit. J. Derm. 48, 21—26 (1936).

BRAIN, R. T., R. C. B. PUGH, and J. A. DUDGEON: Adrenal necrosis in generalized herpes simplex. Arch. Dis. Childh. 32, 120—126 (1957).

BRENNER, S., and R. W. HORNE: A negative staining method for high resolution electron microscopy of viruses. Biochim. biophys. Acta (Amst.) 34, 103—110 (1959).

BRESNICK, E., V. B. THOMPSON, and K. LYMAN: Aggregation of deoxythymidine kinase in dilute solutions: properties of aggregated and disaggregated forms. Arch. Biochem. 114, 352—359 (1966).

BROWN, R. M.: A quantitative study of the inhibition of herpes simplex virus by interferon. Thesis, University of Texas, Austin (1966).

BUDDINGH, G. J., D. I. SCHRUM, J. C. LANIER, and D. J. GUIDRY: Studies of the natural history of herpes simplex infections. Pediatrics 11, 595—610 (1953).

BURGGRAAF, A., et L. F. D. E. LOURENS: Infectieuse-Bulbair-Paralyse (Ziekte van Aujeszky). T. Diergeneesk. 59, 981—1002 (1932). [Abstr. Vet. Bull. (Weybridge) 3, 304 (1932).]

BURNET, F. M.: Virus as Organism. Cambridge, Massachusetts: Harvard University Press. 1945.

BURNET, F. M.: Principles of Animal Virology, 2nd Edition, pp. 246—257. New York: Academic Press. 1960.

BURNET, F. M., and D. LUSH: Herpes Simplex. Studies on the antibody content of human sera. Lancet I, 629—631 (1939a).

BURNET, F. M., and D. LUSH: Studies on experimental herpes infection in mice, using the chorioallantoic technique. J. Path. Bact. 49, 241—259 (1939b).

BURNET, F. M., D. LUSH, and A. V. JACKSON: The relationship of herpes and B viruses: Immunological and epidemiological considerations. Aust. J. exp. Biol. med. Sci. 17, 41—51 (1939).

BURNET, F. M., and S. W. WILLIAMS: Herpes Simplex. A new point of view. Med. J. Aust. 1, 637—642 (1939).

BURNETT, J. W., and S. L. KATZ: A study of the use of 5-iodo-2'-deoxyuridine in cutaneous herpes simplex. J. invest. Derm. **40**, 7—8 (1963).

BURNS, R. P.: A double-blind study of IDU in human herpes simplex keratitis. Arch. Ophthal. **70**, 381—384 (1963).

BUTHALA, D. A.: Cell culture studies on antiviral agents: I. Action of cytosine arabinoside and some comparisons with 5-iodo-2'-deoxyuridine. Proc. Soc. exp. Biol. (N.Y.) **115**, 69—77 (1964).

CAIRNS, H. J. F.: The asynchrony of infection by influenza virus. Virology **3**, 1—14 (1957).

CANELLAKIS, E. S., J. J. JAFFEE, R. MANTSAVINOS, and J. S. KRAKOW: Pyrimidine metabolism. IV. A comparison of normal and regenerating rat liver. J. biol. Chem. **234**, 2096—2099 (1959).

CANTELL, K., and V. TOMMILA: Effect of interferon on experimental vaccinia and herpes simplex virus infections in rabbits' eyes. Lancet **2**, 682—684 (1960).

CARPENTER, C. M., R. A. BOAK, and S. L. WARREN: Symptomatic herpes, a sequela of artificially induced fever. J. exp. Med. **71**, 155—167 (1940).

CARROLL, J. M., E.-M. MARTOLA, P. R. LAIBSON, and C. H. DOHLMAN: The recurrence of herpetic keratitis following iododeoxyuridine therapy. Amer. J. Ophthal. **63**, 103—107 (1967).

CARTON, C. A., and E. D. KILBOURNE: Activation of latent herpes simplex by trigeminal sensory-root section. New Engl. J. Med. **246**, 172—176 (1952).

CASPAR, D. L. D., and A. KLUG: Physical principles in the construction of regular viruses. Cold Spr. Harb. Symp. quant. Biol. **27**, 1—24 (1962).

CECCARELLI, A., e I. DEL MAZZA: Coltura del virus d'Aujeszky su cellule renali di agnello. Zooprofilassi **13**, 159—167 (1958).

CHANGEUX, J.-P.: Allosteric interactions on biosynthetic L-threonine deaminase from *E. coli* K12. Cold Spr. Harb. Symp. quant. Biol. **28**, 497—504 (1963).

CHAPIN, H. B., S. C. WONG, and J. REAPSOME: The value of tissue culture vaccine in the prophylaxis of recurrent attacks of herpetic keratitis. Amer. J. Ophthal. **54**, 255—265 (1962).

CHU, L. W., and G. H. WARREN: Pathogenicity and immunogenicity of herpes simplex virus strains propagated in rabbit kidney tissue. Proc. Soc. exp. Biol. (N.Y.) **105**, 396—399 (1960).

COHEN, S. S.: Growth requirements of bacterial viruses. Bact. Rev. **13**, 1—24 (1949).

COHEN, S. S., J. G. FLAKS, H. D. BARNER, M. R. LOEB, and J. LICHTENSTEIN: The mode of action of 5-fluorouracil and its derivatives. Proc. nat. Acad. Sci. (Wash.) **44**, 1004—1012 (1958).

COLEBATCH, J. H.: Clinical picture of severe generalized viral infection in the newborn. Med. J. Aust. **1**, 377—382 (1955).

COLEMAN, V., and E. JAWETZ: A persistent herpes simplex infection in antibody-free cell culture. Virology **13**, 375—377 (1961).

CORIELL, L. L., G. RAKE, H. BLANK, and T. F. McN. SCOTT: Electron microscopy of herpes simplex. J. Bact. **59**, 61—68 (1950).

CORNER, A. H.: Pathology of experimental Aujeszky's disease in piglets. Res. Vet. Sci. **6**, 337—343 (1965).

COWDRY, E. V.: The problem of intranuclear inclusions in virus diseases. Arch. Path. **18**, 527—542 (1934).

CRANDELL, R. A.: Multiplication and cytopathogenicity of herpes simplex virus in cultures of feline renal cells. Proc. Soc. exp. Biol. (N.Y.) **102**, 508—511 (1959).

CROUSE, H. V., L. L. CORIELL, H. BLANK, and T. F. McN. SCOTT: Cytochemical studies on the intranuclear inclusion of herpes simplex. J. Immunol. **65**, 119—128 (1950).

CSEREY-PECHANY, E., I. BÉLÁDI und G. IVÁNOVICS: Züchtung und Wertmessung des Virus der Aujeszky'schen Krankheit in Gewebekulturen. Acta physiol. Acad. Sci. hung. **2**, 229 (1951).

CSONTOS, L.: To the diagnosis of Aujeszky's disease in pigs. Magy. Állatorv. Lap. **10**, 411—412 (1964).

CSONTOS, L.: Determination of virus content, and possible diagnostic value of organs from pigs died of Aujeszky's disease. Acta vet. Acad. Sci. hung. **16**, 219—222 (1966).

CSONTOS, L., and A. SZÉKY: Gross and microscopic lesions in the nasopharynx of pigs with Aujeszky's disease. Acta vet. Acad. Sci. hung. **16**, 175—186 (1966).

DASCOMB, H. E., C. V. ADAIR, and N. ROGERS: Serologic investigations of herpes simplex virus infections. J. Lab. clin. Med. **46**, 1—11 (1965).

DE DUVE, C.: The lysosome concept. in "Lysosomes", Ciba Foundation Symposium (DE REUCH and CAMERON, eds.), pp. 1—31, Boston-Massachusetts: Little, Brown and Co. 1963.

DELIHAS, N.: The ability of irradiated bacteriophage T 2 to initiate the synthesis of deoxycytidylate hydroxymethylase in *E. coli*. Virology **13**, 242—248 (1961).

DE MAEYER, E., and E. SCHONNE: Starch gel as an overlay for the plaque assay of animal viruses. Virology **24**, 13—18 (1964).

DIRKSEN, M. L., J. S. WIBERG, J. F. KOERNER, and J. M. BUCHANAN: Effect of ultraviolet irradiation of bacteriophage T 2 on enzyme synthesis in host cells. Proc. nat. Acad. Sci. (Wash.) **46**, 1425—1430 (1960).

DODD, K., L. M. JOHNSTON, and G. J. BUDDINGH: Herpetic stomatitis. J. Pediat. **12**, 95—102 (1938).

DOERR, R.: Sitzungsberichte der Gesellschaft der schweizerischen Augenärzte-Diskussion. Klin. Mbl. Augenheilk. **65**, 104 (1920).

DOERR, R.: Der Herpes Febrilis, *in* "Handbuch der Virusforschung" (DOERR und HALLAUER, Hsg.). Vol. 1, pp. 41—45, Wien: Springer-Verlag. 1938.

DOERR, R., und M. KON: Schieneninfektion, Schienenimmunisierung und Konkurrenz der Infektionen im Z.-N.-S. beim Herpes-Virus. Z. Hyg. Infekt.-Kr. **119**, 679—705 (1937).

DOERR, R., und S. SEIDENBERG: Die Konkurrenz von Virusinfektionen im Zentralnervensystem (Phänomen von F. MAGRASSI). Z. Hyg. Infekt.-Kr. **119**, 135—165 (1937).

DOERR, R., et K. VÖCHTING: Études sur le virus de l'herpès fébrile. Rev. gén. Ophthal. (Paris) **34**, 409—421 (1920).

DOW, C., and J. B. MCFERRAN: The pathology of Aujeszky's disease in cattle. J. comp. Path. **72**, 337—347 (1962a).

DOW, C., and J. B. MCFERRAN: The neuropathology of Aujeszky's disease in the pig. Res. Vet. Sci. **3**, 436—442 (1962b).

DUBBS, D. R., and S. KIT: Mutant strains of herpes simplex deficient in thymidine kinase-inducing activity. Virology **22**, 493—502 (1964).

DUBBS, D. R., and S. KIT: The effect of temperature on induction of deoxythymidine kinase activity by herpes simplex mutants. Virology **25**, 256—270 (1965).

DULBECCO, R.: Experiments on photoreactivation of bacteriophages inactivated with ultraviolet irradiation. J. Bact. **59**, 329—347 (1950).

DULBECCO, R.: Photoreactivation, *in* "Radiation Biology" (HOLLAENDER, ed.), vol. II, pp. 455—486, New York: McGraw-Hill Book Co. 1955.

EGGERS, H. J., and I. TAMM: Antiviral chemotherapy. Ann. Rev. Pharmacol. **6**, 231—250 (1966).

EKER, P.: Properties and assay of thymidine deoxyribonucleotide phosphatase of mammalian cells in tissue culture. J. biol. Chem. **240**, 419—422 (1965).

ELFORD, W. J., and I. A. GALLOWAY: The size of the virus of Aujeszky's disease ("pseudorabies", "infectious bulbar paralysis", and "mad itch") by ultrafiltration analysis. J. Hyg. (Lond.) **36**, 532—535 (1936).

ELFORD, W. J., J. R. PERDRAU, and W. SMITH: The filtration of herpes virus through graded collodion membranes. J. Path. Bact. **36**, 49—54 (1933).

ENDERS, J. F.: Bovine amniotic fluid as tissue culture medium in cultivation of poliomyelitis and other viruses. Proc. Soc. exp. Biol. (N.Y.) **82**, 100—105 (1953).

ENGLE, C. G., and R. C. STEWART: Pathogenesis of herpes simplex virus in the rabbit eye. J. Immunol. **92**, 730—733 (1964).

EPSTEIN, M. A.: Observations on the fine structure of mature herpes simplex virus and on the composition of its nucleoid. J. exp. Med. **115**, 1—12 (1962a).

EPSTEIN, M. A.: Observations on the mode of release of herpes virus from infected HeLa cells. J. Cell Biol. **12**, 589—597 (1962b).

EPSTEIN, M. A., K. HUMMELER, and A. BERKALOFF: The entry and distribution of herpes virus and colloidal gold in HeLa cells after contact suspension. J. exp. Med. **119**, 291—302 (1964).

ERIKSON, R. L., and W. SZYBALSKI: The Cs$_2$SO$_4$ equilibrium density gradient and its application for the study of T-even phage DNA: glucosylation and replication. Virology **22**, 11—124 (1964).

ESTEVES, J., and M. R. PINTO: Herpetic urethritis. Brit. J. vener. Dis. **28**, 205—208 (1952).

EVANS, A. S., and J. L. MELNICK: Electron microscope studies of the vesicle and spinal fluids from a case of herpes zoster. Proc. Soc. exp. Biol. (N.Y.) **71**, 283—286 (1949).

EVANS, C. A., H. B. SLAVIN, and G. P. BERRY: The effect of specific antibodies on the progression of virus within the nervous system of young mice. J. exp. Med. **84**, 429—447 (1946).

EY, R. C., W. F. HUGHES, A. W. HOLMES, and F. DEINHARDT: Clinical and laboratory evaluation of iododeoxyuridine (IUD) therapy in herpes simplex keratitis. Arch. Ophthal. **71**, 325—331 (1964).

FALKE, D.: Über die serologischen Beziehungen zwischen B- und Herpes-simplex-Virus in der Komplementbindungsreaktion. Z. Hyg. Infekt.-Kr. **150**, 185—193 (1964).

FALKE, D.: Untersuchungen über die Beziehungen zwischen biologischer Aktivität und Teilchenart bei Herpes-simplex-Virus. Arch. ges. Virusforsch. **15**, 625—639 (1965).

FALKE, D., R. SIEGERT und W. VOGELL: Elektronenmikroskopische Befunde zur Frage der Doppelmembranbildung des Herpes-simplex-Virus. Arch. ges. Virusforsch. **9**, 484—496 (1959).

FARNHAM, A. E.: The formation of microscopic plaques by herpes simplex virus in HeLa cells. Virology **6**, 317—327 (1958).

FARNHAM, A. E., and A. A. NEWTON: The effect of some environmental factors on herpes virus grown in HeLa cells. Virology **7**, 449—461 (1959).

FAUCONNIER, B.: Multiplication du virus des oreillons, du virus de la vaccine, et du virus de l'herpès sur cellules de rein de tortue (Testudo graeca) cultivées suivant une méthode simplifiée. Ann. Inst. Pasteur **105**, 439—444 (1963).

FELGENHAUER, K., und A. STAMMLER: Die histochemisch nachweisbaren Veränderungen in der mit dem Virus des Herpes simplex inokulierten Zellkultur. Arch. ges. Virusforsch. **12**, 223—232 (1962).

FELLUGA, B.: Electron microscopic observations on pseudorabies virus development in a line of pig kidney cells. Ann. Sclavo **5**, 412—424 (1963).

FELTON, F. G., and L. V. SCOTT: Studies on hemagglutination with herpes simplex virus. II. The factors involved in the technique. J. Immunol. **86**, 42—49 (1961).

FERNANDEZ, C. G.: Persistence of herpes simplex virus in HeLa cells. Nature (Lond.) **185**, 268 (1960).

FIALA, S., A. FIALA, G. TOBAR, and H. McQUILLA: Deoxynucleotidase activity in rat liver and certain tumors. J. nat. Cancer Inst. **28**, 1269—1289 (1962).

FIELD, E. J.: Pathogenesis of herpetic encephalitis following corneal and masseteric inoculation. J. Path. Bact. **64**, 1—11 (1952).

FINDLAY, G. M., and F. O. MACCALLUM: Recurrent traumatic herpes. Lancet **238**, 259—261 (1940).

FISHER, T. N., and E. FISHER, JR.: Effects of cortisone and herpes simplex virus on metabolic processes. I. Alterations in HeLa cell metabolism. Proc. Soc. exp. Biol. (N.Y.) **100**, 780—786 (1959).

FISHER, T. N., and E. FISHER, JR.: Host metabolic alterations following herpes simplex infection. Virology **13**, 308—314 (1961).

FITZGERALD, J. E., and L. E. HANSON: A comparison of some properties of laryngotracheitis and herpes simplex viruses. Amer. J. vet. Res. **24**, 1297—1303 (1963).

FLANAGAN, J. F.: Hydrolytic enzymes in KB cells infected with poliovirus and herpes simplex virus. J. Bact. **91**, 789—797 (1966).

FLANAGAN, J. F.: Virus-specific ribonucleic acid synthesis in KB cells infected with herpes simplex virus. J. Virol. 1, 583—590 (1967).

FLORMAN, A. L., and R. L. MINDLIN: Generalized herpes simplex in an eleven-day-old premature infant. Amer. J. Dis. Child. 83, 481—486 (1952).

FLORMAN, A., and F. W. TRADER: A comparative study of pathogenicity and antigenicity of four strains of herpes simplex. J. Immunol. 55, 263—275 (1947).

FOERSTER, D. W., and L. V. SCOTT: Herpes simplex-Stevens-Johnson syndrome. Isolation of herpes simplex virus from a patient with erythema multiforme exudativum (Stevens-Johnson-syndrome). New Engl. J. Med. 259, 473—475 (1958).

FORCE, E. E., R. C. STEWART, and R. F. HAFF: Herpes simplex skin infection in rabbits. I. Effect of 5-iodo-2'-deoxyuridine. Virology 23, 363—369 (1964).

FORCE, E. E., R. C. STEWART, and R. F. HAFF: Development of interferon in rabbit dermis after infection with herpes simplex virus. Virology 25, 322—325 (1965).

FRANK, S. B.: Formolized herpes virus therapy and the neutralizing substance in herpes simplex. J. invest. Derm. 1, 267—282 (1938).

FREARSON, P. M., S. KIT, and D. R. DUBBS: Deoxythymidylate synthetase and deoxythymidine kinase activities of virus-infected animal cells. Cancer Res. 25, 737—744 (1965).

FREARSON, P. M., S. KIT, and D. R. DUBBS: Induction of dihydrofolate reductase activity by SV40 and polyoma virus. Cancer Res. 26, 1653—1660 (1966).

FREIFELDER, D., and P. F. DAVISON: Physicochemical studies on the reaction between formaldehyde and DNA. Biophys. J. 3, 49—63 (1963).

FREUNDLICH, M., and H. E. UMBARGER: The effects of analogues of threonine and of isoleucine on the properties of threonine deaminase. Cold Spr. Harb. Symp. quant. Biol. 28, 505—511 (1963).

FRUITSTONE, M. J., G. H. WADDELL, and M. M. SIGEL: An interferon produced in response to infection by herpes simplex virus. Proc. Soc. exp. Biol. (N.Y.) 117, 804—807 (1964).

FUJIWARA, S., and A. S. KAPLAN: Site of protein synthesis in cells infected with pseudorabies virus. Virology 32, 60—68 (1967).

GALLOWAY, I. A.: Aujeszky's disease. Vet. Rec. 50, 745—762 (1938).

GARABEDIAN, G. A., and J. T. SYVERTON: Studies on herpes simplex virus. I. An antigenic analysis of four strains of virus isolated from a human subject. J. infect. Dis. 96, 1—13 (1955).

GÉDER, L., L. VÁCZI, and M. KOLLER: Persistent varicella and herpes simplex virus infection of a continuous monkey kidney cell culture. Acta virol. 9, 431—436 (1965).

GERHARDT, J. C., and A. B. PARDEE: The effect of the feedback inhibition, CTP, on subunit interactions in aspartate transcarbamylase. Cold Spr. Harb. Symp. quant. Biol. 28, 491—496 (1963).

GLASGOW, L. A., and K. HABEL: The role of interferon in vaccinia virus infection of mouse embryo tissue culture. J. exp. Med. 115, 503—512 (1962).

GLASGOW, L. A., and K. HABEL: Role of polyoma virus and interferon in a herpes simplex virus infection in vitro. Virology 19, 328—339 (1963).

GLOVER, R. E.: Cultivation of the virus of Aujeszky's disease on the chorioallantoic membrane of the developing egg. Brit. J. exp. Path. 20, 150—158 (1939).

GOLD, E., P. WILDY, and D. H. WATSON: The development of infectivity, antigens and particles in herpes infected cells. J. Immunol. 91, 666—669 (1963).

GOLD, J. A., R. C. STEWART, and J. McKEE: The epidemiology and chemotherapy of herpes simplex keratitis and herpes simplex skin infections. Ann. N.Y. Acad. Sci. 130, 209—212 (1965).

GOOD, R. A., and B. CAMPBELL: Potentiating effect of anaphylactic and histamine shock upon herpes simplex virus infection in rabbits. Proc. Soc. exp. Biol. (N.Y.) 59, 305—306 (1945).

GOOD, R. A., and B. CAMPBELL: Precipitation of latent Herpes simplex encephalitis by anaphylactic shock. Proc. Soc. exp. Biol. (N.Y.) 68, 82—87 (1948).

GOODPASTURE, E. W.: The axis-cylinder of peripheral nerves as portals of entry to the central nervous system for the virus of herpes simplex in experimentally infected rabbits. Amer. J. Path. 1, 11—28 (1925a).

GOODPASTURE, E. W.: The pathways of infection of the central nervous system in herpetic encephalitis of rabbits contracted by contact; with a comparative comment on medullary lesions in a case of human poliomyelitis. Amer. J. Path. 1, 29—46 (1925b).

GOODPASTURE, E. W., and O. TEAGUE: Transmission of herpes febrilis along nerves in experimentally infected rabbits. J. med. Res. 44, 139—184 (1923).

GORDON, W. A. M., and D. LUKE: An outbreak of Aujeszky's disease in swine with a heavy mortality in piglets, illness in sows and deaths in utero. Vet. Rec. 67, 591—597 (1955).

GRAY, A., and T. F. McN. SCOTT: Some observations on the intracellular localization of the virus of herpes simplex in the chick embryo liver. J. exp. Med. 100, 473—484 (1954).

GRAY, A., T. TOKUMARU, and T. F. McN. SCOTT: Different cytopathogenic effects observed in HeLa cells infected with herpes simplex virus. Arch. ges. Virusforsch. 8, 59—76 (1958).

GRESSER, I., and J. F. ENDERS: The effect of trypsin on representative myxoviruses. Virology 13, 420—426 (1961).

GRÜTER, W.: Experimentelle und klinische Untersuchungen über den sogenannten Herpes corneae. Ber. Dtsch. ophthal. Ges. 42, 162—167 (1920).

GUSTAFSON, D. P., and J. R. SAUNDERS: Pseudorabies virus in swine: a new virulent strain. Fed. Proc. 25, 421 (1966).

HALE, B. D., R. C. RENDTORFF, L. C. WALKER, and A. N. ROBERTS: Epidemic herpetic stomatitis in an orphanage nursery. J. Amer. med. Ass. 183, 1068—1072 (1963).

HALLAUER, C.: Über die Immunisierung des Zentralnervensystems mit einem nicht-encephalitogenen Herpesstamm. Z. Hyg. Infekt.-Kr. 119, 213—224 (1937).

HAMADA, C., T. KAMIYA, and A. S. KAPLAN: Serological analysis of some enzymes present in pseudorabies virus-infected and noninfected cells. Virology 28, 271—281 (1966).

HAMADA, C., and A. S. KAPLAN: Kinetics of synthesis of various types of antigenic proteins in cells infected with pseudorabies virus. J. Bact. 89, 1328—1334 (1965).

HAMAR, M.: Über die Varianten des Herpesvirus hominis. Arch. klin. exp. Derm. 220, 283—289 (1964).

HAMBURG, V. P., and G. J. SVET-MOLDAVSKY: Artificial heterogenization of tumors by means of herpes simplex and polyoma viruses. Nature (Lond.) 203, 772—773 (1964).

HAMPAR, B.: Persistent cyclic herpes simplex virus infection in vitro. II. Localization of virus, degree of cell destruction, and mechanisms of virus transmission. III. Asynchrony in the progression of infection and cell growth. J. Bact. 91, 1959—1964; 1965—1970 (1966a and b).

HAMPAR, B., and M. L. COPELAND: Persistent herpes simplex virus infection in vitro with cycles of cell destruction and regrowth. J. Bact. 90, 205—212 (1965).

HAMPAR, B., and S. A. ELLISON: Chromosomal aberrations induced by an animal virus. Nature (Lond.) 192, 145—147 (1961).

HAMPAR, B., and S. A. ELLISON: Cellular alterations in the MCH line of chinese hamster cells following infection with herpes simplex virus. Proc. nat. Acad. Sci. (Wash.) 49, 474—480 (1963).

HAMPAR, B., and M. A. KEEHN: Cumulative changes in the antigenic properties of herpes simplex virus from persistently infected cell cultures. J. Immunol. 99, 554—557 (1967).

HANCOCK, B. B., E. H. BOHL, and J. M. BIRKELAND: Swine kidney cultures. Susceptibility to viruses, and use in isolation of enteric viruses of swine. Amer. J. vet. Res. 20, 127—132 (1959).

HANNA, C., and K. P. WILKINSON: Effect of iododeoxyuridine on the uptake of tritium-labeled thymidine in the rabbit cornea infected with herpes simplex. Exp. Eye Res. 4, 31—35 (1965).

HANSON, R. P.: The history of pseudorabies in the United States. J. Amer. vet. Med. Ass. **124**, 259—261 (1954).

HART, D. R. L., V. J. F. BRIGHTMAN, G. G. READSHAW, G. PORTER, and M. J. TULLY: Treatment of herpes keratitis with IDU. Arch. Ophthal. **73**, 623—634 (1965).

HAY, J., G. J. KÖTELES, H. M. KEIR, and H. SUBAK-SHARPE: Herpes virus specified ribonucleic acids. Nature (Lond.) **210**, 387—390 (1966).

HAYWARD, M. E.: Serological studies with herpes simplex virus. Brit. J. exp. Path. **30**, 520—529 (1949).

HAYWARD, M. E.: Serological diagnosis of herpes simplex infections. Lancet **1**, 856—858 (1950).

HENOCQ, E., J. DE RUDDER, J. MAURIN et P. LÉPINE: Essai de thérapeutique de l'herpès récidivant par un vaccin préparé en culture cellulaire et inactivé par les rayons ultra-violets. II. Essais cliniques. Sem. Hôp. (Paris) **40**, 1474—1480 (1964).

HERRIOTT, R. M.: Infectious nucleic acids, a new dimension in virology. Science **134**, 256—260 (1961).

HERSHEY, A. D.: Chemistry and viral growth. in "Currents of Biochemical Research", pp. 1—28, New York: Interscience. 1956.

HINZE, H. C., and D. L. WALKER: Occurrence of focal three-dimensional proliferation in cultured human cells after prolonged infection with herpes simplex virus. J. exp. Med. **113**, 885—898 (1961a).

HINZE, H. C., and D. L. WALKER: Variation of herpes simplex virus in persistently infected tissue cultures. J. Bact. **82**, 498—504 (1961b).

HO, M., and J. R. ENDERS: Further studies on an inhibitor of viral activity appearing in infected cell cultures and its role in chronic viral infections. Virology **9**, 446—447 (1959).

HOGGAN, M. D., and B. ROIZMAN: The effect of temperature of incubation on the formation and release of herpes simplex virus in infected FL cells. Virology **8**, 508—524 (1959a).

HOGGAN, M. D., and B. ROIZMAN: The isolation and properties of a variant of herpes simplex producing multinucleated giant cells in monolayer cultures in the presence of antibody. Amer. J. Hyg. **70**, 208—219 (1959b).

HOGGAN, M. D., B. ROIZMAN, and P. R. ROANE, JR.: Further studies of variants of herpes simplex virus that produce syncytia or pock-like lesions in cell culture. Amer. J. Hyg. **73**, 114—122 (1961).

HOLDEN, M.: The nature and property of the virus of herpes. J. infect. Dis. **50**, 218—236 (1932).

HOLMES, I. H., and D. H. WATSON: An electron microscope study of the attachment and penetration of herpes virus in BHK21 cells. Virology **21**, 112—123 (1963).

HOLZEL, A., G. V. FELDMAN, J, O'H. TOBIN, and J. HARPER: Herpes Simplex. A study of complement-fixing antibodies at different ages. Acta paediat. (Uppsala) **42**, 206—214 (1953).

HORNE, R. W., and P. WILDY: Symmetry in virus architecture. Virology **15**, 348—373 (1961).

HOWES, D. W.: The growth of poliovirus in cultured cells. III. The asynchronous response of HeLa cells multiply infected with type I poliovirus. Virology **9**, 110—126 (1959).

HSU, T. C., and C. E. SOMERS: Effect of 5-bromodeoxyuridine on mammalian chromosomes. Proc. nat. Acad. Sci. (Wash.) **47**, 396—403 (1961).

HUANG, A. S., and R. R. WAGNER: Penetration of herpes simplex virus into human epidermoid cells. Proc. Soc. exp. Biol. (N.Y.) **116**, 863—869 (1964).

HULL, R. N., and F. B. PECK, JR.: Vaccination against herpesvirus infections. First International Conference on Vaccines against Viral and Rickettsial Diseases of Man. pp. 266—275. Wld Hlth Org., Washington, D. C. (1967).

HURST, E. W.: Studies on pseudorabies (infectious bulbar paralysis, mad itch). I. Histology of the disease, with a note on the symptomatology. J. exp. Med. **58**, 415—431 (1933).

HURST, E. W.: Studies on pseudorabies (infectious bulbar paralysis, mad itch). II. Routes of infection in the rabbit, with remarks on the relation of the virus to other viruses affecting the nervous system. J. exp. Med. **59**, 729—749 (1934).

HURST, E. W.: Studies on pseudorabies (infectious bulbar paralysis, mad itch). III. The disease in the rhesus monkey, Macaca mulatta. J. exp. Med. **63**, 449—463 (1936).

ISAACS, A.: Nature and function of interferon. *in* "Perspectives in Virology" (POLLARD, ed.), Vol. II, pp. 117—123, Minneapolis: Burgess Publishing Co. 1961.

ISAACS, A., D. C. BURKE, and L. FADEEVA: Effect of interferon on the growth of viruses on the chick chorion. Brit. J. exp. Path. **39**, 447—458 (1958).

ISAACS, A., and J. LINDENMANN: Virus interference. I. The interferon. Proc. roy. Soc. B **147**, 258—267 (1957).

IVANIČOVÁ, S.: Inactivation of Aujeszky disease (pseudorabies) by fluorocarbon. Acta virol. **5**, 328 (1961).

IVANIČOVÁ, S., R. ŠKODA, V. MAYER, and F. SOKOL: Inactivation of Aujeszky disease (pseudorabies) virus by nitrous acid. Acta virol. **7**, 7—15 (1963).

IVÁNOVICS, G., I. BÉLÁDI, and E. SZÖLLÖSY: Interference between variants of pseudorabies virus demonstrable in tissue culture. Nature (Lond.) **176**, 972 (1955 a).

IVÁNOVICS, G., I. BÉLÁDI, and E. SZÖLLÖSY: Variation of the cytopathogenic activity of Aujeszky disease (pseudorabies) virus. Acta microbiol. Acad. Sci. hung. **III**, 159—172 (1955 b).

JAGGER, J.: Photoreactivation. Bact. Rev. **22**, 99—142 (1958).

JANOWSKI, H., and H. OBERFELD: Aujeszky's disease in Poland. Bull. Off. int. Epiz. **63**, 1853—1864 (1965).

JAWETZ, E., M. F. ALLENDE, and V. R. COLEMAN: Studies on herpes simplex virus. VI. Observations on patients with recurrent herpetic lesions injected with herpes viruses or their antigens. Amer. J. med. Sci. **229**, 477—485 (1955).

JAWETZ, E., V. COLEMAN, and M. F. ALLENDE: Studies on herpes simplex virus. II. A soluble antigen of herpes virus possessing skin-reactive properties. J. Immunol. **67**, 197—205 (1951).

JAWETZ, E., V. R. COLEMAN, and E. R. MERRILL: Studies on herpes simplex virus. VII. Immunological comparison of strains of herpes simplex. J. Immunol. **75**, 28—34 (1955).

JAWETZ, E., M. OKUMOTO, and M. SONNE: Studies on herpes simplex. X. The effect of corticosteroids on herpetic keratitis in the rabbit. J. Immunol. **83**, 486—490 (1959).

JENEY, E., É. GÖNCZÖL, and L. VÁCZI: Replication of herpes simplex virus in arginine-free media. I. Effect of arginine-deficiency in different tissue culture cells. Acta microbiol. Acad. Sci. hung. **14**, 31—37 (1967).

JEPSON, C. N.: Treatment of herpes simplex of the cornea with IDU: a double-blind study. Amer. J. Ophthal. **57**, 213—217 (1964).

JOHNSON, R. T.: The pathogenesis of herpes virus encephalitis. I. Virus pathways to the nervous system of suckling mice by fluorescent antibody staining. J. exp. Med. **119**, 343—356 (1964 a).

JOHNSON, R. T.: The pathogenesis of herpes virus encephalitis: II. A cellular basis for the development of resistance with age. J. exp. Med. **120**, 359—374 (1964 b).

JURETIC, M.: Incubation period of primary herpetic infection. Helv. paediat. Acta **15**, 102—107 (1960).

KAMIYA, T., T. BEN-PORAT, and A. S. KAPLAN: The role of progeny viral DNA in the regulation of enzyme and DNA synthesis. Biochem. biophys. Res. Commun. **16**, 410—415 (1964).

KAMIYA, T., T. BEN-PORAT, and A. S. KAPLAN: Control of certain aspects of the infective process by progeny viral DNA. Virology **26**, 577—589 (1965).

KANAZAWA, K.: Y a-t-il une relation immunologique entre le virus vaccinal et le virus herpétique? Expériences sur la souris. Jap. J. exp. Med. **16**, 109—115 (1938).

KAPLAN, A. S.: A study of the herpes simplex virus-rabbit kidney cell system by the plaque technique. Virology **4**, 435—457 (1957).

KAPLAN, A. S.: Analysis of the intracellular development of a DNA-containing mammalian virus (pseudorabies) by means of ultraviolet light irradiation. Virology **16**, 305–313 (1962).

KAPLAN, A. S.: Studies on the replicating pool of viral DNA in cells infected with pseudorabies virus. Virology **24**, 19–25 (1964).

KAPLAN, A. S., and T. BEN-PORAT: The effect of pseudorabies virus on the nucleic acid metabolism and on the nuclei of rabbit kidney cells. Virology **8**, 352–366 (1959).

KAPLAN, A. S., and T. BEN-PORAT: The incorporation of C^{14}-labeled nucleosides into rabbit kidney cells infected with pseudorabies virus. Virology **11**, 12–27 (1960).

KAPLAN, A. S., and T. BEN-PORAT: The action of 5-fluorouracil on the nucleic acid metabolism of pseudorabies virus-infected and noninfected rabbit kidney cells. Virology **13**, 78–92 (1961).

KAPLAN, A. S., and T. BEN-PORAT: The pattern of viral and cellular DNA synthesis in pseudorabies virus-infected cells in the logarithmic phase of growth. Virology **19**, 205–214 (1963).

KAPLAN, A. S., and T. BEN-PORAT: Mode of replication of pseudorabies virus DNA. Virology **23**, 90–95 (1964).

KAPLAN, A. S., and T. BEN-PORAT: Mode of antiviral action of 5-iodouracil deoxyriboside. J. molec. Biol. **19**, 320–332 (1966a).

KAPLAN, A. S., and T. BEN-PORAT: The replication of the double-stranded DNA of an animal virus during intracellular multiplication. 9th International Congress for Microbiology, Symposia, pp. 463–482 (1966b).

KAPLAN, A. S., and T. BEN-PORAT: Differential incorporation of iododeoxyuridine into the DNA of pseudorabies virus-infected and noninfected cells. Virology **31**, 734–736 (1967a).

KAPLAN, A. S., and T. BEN-PORAT: Effect of nucleoside analogues on cells infected with pseudorabies virus. 2nd International Symp. Applied and Medical Virology, Sanders and Lennette, eds.), pp. 56–76, St. Louis: Warren H. Green, Inc. (1967b).

KAPLAN, A. S., T. BEN-PORAT, and C. COTO: Studies on the control of the infective process in cells infected with pseudorabies virus. *in* "Molecular Biology of Viruses" (COLTER and PARANCHYCH, eds.), pp. 527–545, New York: Academic Press. 1967.

KAPLAN, A. S., T. BEN-PORAT, and T. KAMIYA: Incorporation of 5-bromodeoxyuridine and 5-iododeoxyuridine into viral DNA and its effect on the infective process. Ann. N.Y. Acad. Sci. **130**, 226–239 (1965).

KAPLAN, A. S., and A. E. VATTER: A comparison of herpes simplex and pseudorabies viruses. Virology **7**, 394–407 (1959).

KAPSENBERG, J. G.: Possible antigenic relationship between varicella-zoster virus and herpes simplex virus. Arch. ges. Virusforsch. **15**, 67–73 (1964).

KAUFMAN, H. E.: The diagnosis of corneal herpes simplex by fluorescent antibody staining. Arch. Ophthal. **64**, 382–384 (1960).

KAUFMAN, H. E.: Clinical cure of herpes simplex keratitis by 5-iodo-2'-deoxyuridine. Proc. Soc. exp. Biol. (N.Y.) **109**, 251–252 (1962).

KAUFMAN, H. E.: *In vivo* studies with antiviral agents. Ann. N.Y. Acad. Sci. **130**, 168–180 (1965).

KAUFMAN, H. E., D. C. BROWN, and E. M. ELLISON: Recurrent herpes in the rabbit and man. Science **156**, 1628–1629 (1967).

KAUFMAN, H. E., J. A. CAPELLA, E. D. MALONEY, J. E. ROBBINS, G. M. COOPER, and M. H. UOTILA: Corneal toxicity of cytosine arabinoside. Arch. Ophthal. **72**, 535–540 (1964).

KAUFMAN, H. E., and C. HEIDELBERGER: Therapeutic antiviral action of 5-trifluoromethyl-2'-deoxyuridine in herpes simplex keratitis. Science **145**, 585–586 (1964).

KAUFMAN, H. E., A. B. NESBURN, and E. D. MALONEY: IDU therapy of herpes simplex. Arch. Ophthal. **67**, 583–591 (1962).

KEIR, H. M., and E. GOLD: Deoxyribonucleic acid nucleotidyltransferase and deoxyribonuclease from cultured cells infected with herpes simplex virus. Biochim. biophys. Acta (Amst.) **72**, 263—276 (1963).

KEIR, H. M., J. HAY, J. M. MORRISON, and H. SUBAK-SHARPE: Altered properties of deoxyribonucleic acid nucleotidyltransferase after infection of mammalian cells with herpes simplex virus. Nature (Lond.) **210**, 369—371 (1966a).

KEIR, H. M., H. SUBAK-SHARPE, W. I. H. SHEDDEN, D. H. WATSON, and P. WILDY: Immunological evidence for a specific DNA polymerase produced after infection by herpes simplex virus. Virology **30**, 154—157 (1966b).

KELLENBERGER, E.: The physical state of the bacterial nucleus. 10th Symp. Soc. gen. Microbiol. pp. 39—65 (1960).

KENT, T. H., and D. P. NICHOLSON: Herpes simplex encephalitis. Amer. J. Dis. Child. **108**, 644—647 (1964).

KERN, A. B., and B. L. SCHIFF: Vaccine therapy in recurrent herpes simplex. Arch. Derm. **89**, 844—845 (1964).

KERSTING, G., B. KERÉKJARTÓ und B. ROHDE: Über charakteristische Zellveränderungen in der Kultur epithelialen Gewebes nach der Infektion mit Aujeszky- und B-Virus. Z. Naturforsch. **13b**, 158—164 (1958).

KILBOURNE, E., and F. L. HORSFALL, Jr.: Studies of herpes simplex virus in newborn mice. J. Immunol. **67**, 321—329 (1951).

KING, L. S.: Experimental encephalitis. Some factors affecting infection with certain neurotropic viruses. J. exp. Med. **72**, 573—593 (1940).

KIT, S., and D. R. DUBBS: Acquisition of thymidine kinase activity by herpes simplex infected mouse fibroblast cells. Biochem. biophys. Res. Commun. **11**, 55—59 (1963a).

KIT, S., and D. R. DUBBS: Non-functional thymidine kinase cistron in bromodeoxyuridine resistant strains of herpes simplex virus. Biochem. biophys. Res. Commun. **13**, 500—504 (1963b).

KIT, S., and D. R. DUBBS: Properties of deoxythymidine kinase partially purified from noninfected and virus-infected mouse fibroblast cells. Virology **26**, 16—27 (1965).

KIT, S., D. R. DUBBS, and M. ANKEN: Altered properties of thymidine kinase after infection of mouse fibroblast cells with herpes simplex virus. J. Virol. **1**, 238—240 (1967).

KIT, S., D. R. DUBBS, and P. M. FREARSON: Enzymes of nucleic acid metabolism in cells infected with polyoma virus. Cancer Res. **26**, 638—646 (1966).

KIT, S., D. R. DUBBS, P. M. FREARSON, and J. L. MELNICK: Enzyme induction in SV40 infected green monkey kidney cultures. Virology **29**, 69—83 (1966).

KLEMPERER, H. G., G. R. HAYNES, W. I. H. SHEDDEN, and D. H. WATSON: A virus-specific thymidine kinase in BHK 21 cells infected with herpes simplex virus. Virology **31**, 120—128 (1967).

KLUG, A., and O. L. D. CASPAR: Structure of small viruses. Advanc. Virus Res. **7**, 225—325 (1960).

KOBAYASHI, S., and T. NAKAMURA: Herpes corneae and IDU development of IDU resistance in herpes simplex virus. Jap. J. Ophthal. **8**, 14—20 (1964).

KOHLHAGE, H.: Differenzierung von Plaquevarianten des Herpes-simplex-Virus durch Gradientenzentrifugierung und Säulenchromatographie. Zbl. Bakt. I. Abt. Orig. **191**, 252—256 (1963/64).

KOHLHAGE, H.: Differenzierung von Plaquevarianten des Herpes-simplex-Virus durch Gradientenzentrifugation und Säulenchromatographie. Arch. ges. Virusforsch. **14**, 358—365 (1964).

KOHLHAGE, H., und G. SCHIEFERSTEIN: Untersuchungen über die genetische Stabilität des Plaquebildes beim Herpes-simplex-Virus in Zellkulturen. Arch. ges. Virusforsch. **15**, 640—650 (1965).

KOHLHAGE, H., und R. SIEGERT: Zwei genetisch determinierte Varianten eines Herpes-simplex-Stammes. Arch. ges. Virusforsch. **12**, 273—286 (1962).

KOJNOK, J.: Mother's milk and the spread of Aujeszky's disease in sucking pigs. Acta vet. Acad. Sci. hung. **7**, 273—276 (1957).

KOJNOK, J.: The role of pigs in the spreading of Aujeszky's disease among cattle and sheep. Acta vet. Acad. Sci. hung. **12**, 53—58 (1962).

KOJNOK, J.: The role of carrier sows in the spread of Aujeszky's disease to suckling pigs. Data on Aujeszky's virus carriership among fattening pigs. Acta vet. Acad. Sci. hung. **15**, 283—295 (1965).

KOJNOK, J., and E. GRÉCZI: Serum against Aujeszky's disease in sucking pigs. Acta vet. Acad. Sci. hung. **7**, 423—427 (1957).

KOJNOK, J., and J. SURJAN: Investigations concerning the colostral immunity of pigs in cases of Aujeszky's disease. Acta vet. Acad. Sci. hung. **13**, 111—118 (1963).

LAIBSON, P. R., and S. KIBRICK: Reactivation of herpetic keratitis by epinephrine in rabbit. Arch. Ophthal. **75**, 254—260 (1966).

LAIBSON, P. R., and J. H. LEOPOLD: An evaluation of double-blind IDU therapy in 100 cases of herpetic keratitis. Trans. Amer. Acad. Ophthal. Otolaryng. **68**, 22—34 (1964).

LAMONT, H. G.: Observations on Aujeszky's disease in Northern Ireland. Vet. Rec. **58**, 621—625 (1946).

LAMONT, H. G., and W. A. M. GORDON: Aujeszky's disease — a sporadic case in a fox terrier bitch. Vet. Rec. **62**, 596 (1950).

LAMPSON, G. P., A. A. TYTELL, M. M. NEMES, and M. R. HILLEMAN: Characterization of chick embryo interferon produced by a DNA virus. Proc. Soc. exp. Biol. (N.Y.) **118**, 441—448 (1965).

LANDO, D., J. DE RUDDER et M. PRIVAT DE GARILHE: A propos de la composition du DNA du virus herpétique. Bull. Soc. Chim. biol. (Paris) **67**, 1033—1042 (1965).

LAUDA, E., und P. REZEK: Zur Histopathologie des Herpes Simplex. Virchows Arch. path. Anat. **262**, 827—837 (1926).

LEBRUN, J.: Cellular localization of herpes simplex virus by means of fluorescent antibody. Virology **2**, 496—510 (1956).

LEIDER, W., R. L. MAGOFFIN, E. H. LENNETTE, and L. N. R. LEONARDS: Herpes simplex virus encephalitis — its possible association with reactivated latent infection. New Engl. J. Med. **273**, 341—347 (1965).

LENNETTE, E. H., and H. KOPROWSKI: Influence of age on the susceptibility of mice to infection with certain neurotropic viruses. J. Immunol. **49**, 175—191 (1944).

LEOPOLD, I. H.: Recent advances in ocular therapy. in "The Year Book of Ophthalmology" 1962—63 Ser: 5. Year Book Med. Publ., Chicago, Illinois (1963).

LEOPOLD, I. H.: Clinical experience with nucleosides in herpes simplex eye infections in man and animals. Ann. N. Y. Acad. Sci. **130**, 181—191 (1965).

LEOPOLD, I. H., and T. W. SERY: Epidemiology of herpes simplex keratitis. Invest. Ophthal. **2**, 498—503 (1963).

LÉPINE, P., F. ARTZET et G. CEOLIN: Conservation du virus herpétique. Ann. Inst. Pasteur **98**, 750—753 (1960).

LÉPINE, P., J. DE RUDDER, J. MAURIN et E. HENOCQ: Essai de thérapeutique de l'herpès récidivant par un vaccin préparé en culture cellulaire et inactivé par les rayons ultra-violets. I. Préparation du vaccin et essais d'immunisation sur l'animal. Sem. Hôp. Paris **40**, 1471—1474 (1964).

LEVADITI, C.: Association entre ultravirus. Herpès et rage des rues. C. R. Soc. Biol. (Paris) **136**, 331—332 (1942).

LEVADITI, C., et P. HARVIER: Le virus de l'encéphalite léthargique (encéphalite épidémique). C. R. Soc. Biol. (Paris) **83**, 354—355 (1920).

LEVADITI, C., G. HORNUS et P. HABER: Virulence de l'ultravirus herpétique administré par voies nasale et digestive. Mécanisme de sa neuroprobasie centripète. Ann. Inst. Pasteur **54**, 389—420 (1935).

LEVADITI, C., et L. REINIE: Association persistante, quoique reductible, du virus vaccinal et du virus de l'herpès. C. R. Soc. Biol. (Paris) **134**, 378—382 (1940).

LEWIS, V. J., Jr., and L. V. SCOTT: Nutritional requirements for the production of herpes simplex virus. I. Influence of glucose and glutamine on herpes simplex virus production by HeLa cells. J. Bact. **83**, 475—482 (1962).

LIPSCHÜTZ, B.: Untersuchungen über die Ätiologie der Krankheiten der Herpesgruppe (Herpes zoster, Herpes genitalis, Herpes febrilis). Arch. Derm. Syph. (Berl.) **136**, 428—482 (1921).

LITTLEFIELD, J. W.: Studies on thymidine kinase in cultured mouse fibroblasts. Biochim. biophys. Acta (Amst.) **95**, 14—22 (1965).

LOVE, R., and P. WILDY: Cytochemical studies of the nucleoproteins of HeLa cells infected with herpes virus. J. Cell Biol. **17**, 237—254 (1963).

LÖWENSTEIN, A.: Ätiologische Untersuchungen über den fieberhaften Herpes. Münch. med. Wschr. **66**, 769—770 (1919).

LUKASHOV, I. I., and V. S. NIKITIN: Prophylactic and therapeutic effects of gamma globulin in Aujeszky's disease. Veterinariya **35**, 48—50 (in Russian) (1958).

LUNTZ, M. H., and F. O. McCALLUM: Treatment of herpes simplex keratitis with 5-iodo-2′-deoxyuridine. Brit. J. Ophthal. **47**, 449—456 (1963).

LURIA, S. E.: Radiation and viruses. In "Radiation Biology" (HOLLAENDER, ed.), Vol. II, p. 333. New York: McGraw-Hill Book Company. 1955.

LURIA, S. E., and R. LATARJET: Ultraviolet irradiation of bacteriophage during intracellular growth. J. Bact. **53**, 149—163 (1947).

LUSE, S., P. FRIEDMAN, and M. SMITH: An ultrastructural study of herpes simplex encephalitis. Amer. J. Path. **46**, 8a (1965).

LWOFF, A., R. DULBECCO, M. VOGT, and M. LWOFF: Kinetics of the release of poliomyelitis virus from single cells. Virology **1**, 128—139 (1955).

MacCALLUM, F. O.: Generalized herpes simplex in the neonatal period. Acta virol. **3** (Suppl.), 17—21 (1959).

MAGRASSI, F.: Studii sull'infezione e sull'immunità da virus erpetico. II. Sul contenuto in virus del cervello, in raporto a diversi ceppi di virus, a diverse vie d'infezione, a diversi fasi del processo infettivo. III. Rapporti tra infezione e superinfezione di fronte ai processi immunitari: sulla possibilità di profondamente modificare il decorso e gli esiti del processo infettivo già in atto. Z. Hyg. Infekt.-Kr. **117**, 501—528, 573—620 (1935—1936).

MALEY, F., and G. F. MALEY: IV. Activities of deoxycytidylate deaminase and thymidylate synthetase in normal rat liver and hepatomas. Cancer Res. **21**, 1421—1426 (1961).

MANNINGER, R., et J. MÓCZY: Traité des maladies internes des animaux domestiques. Paris: Vigot Frères, pp. 457—464 (1959).

MAREK, J.: Klinische Mitteilungen. Z. Tiermed. **8**, 389—392 (1904).

MARINESCO, G., et S. DRAGANESCO: Recherches expérimentales sur le neurotropism du virus herpétique. Ann. Inst. Pasteur **37**, 753—783 (1923).

MARTIN, N., e D. CANEJA: Tratamiento biologico del herpes ocular. Arch. Ottal. **33**, 367 (1933).

MAŠIĆ, M., M. ERCEGAN und M. PETROVIČ: Die Bedeutung der Tonsillen für die Pathogenese und Diagnose der Aujeszky'schen Krankheit bei Schweinen. Zbl. Vet.-Med. **12**, 398—405 (1965).

MAYER, V., and R. SKODA: The behaviour of modified and virulent strains of pseudorabies (Aujeszky disease) virus at different temperatures. Acta virol. **6**, 95 (1962).

MAZZONE, H. M., and G. YERGANIAN: Gross and chromosomal cytology of virus infected Chinese hamster cells. Exp. Cell Res. **30**, 591—592 (1963).

McAUSLAN, B. R., P. HERDE, D. PETT, and J. ROSS: Nucleases of virus-infected animal cells. Biochem. biophys. Res. Commun. **20**, 586—591 (1965).

McFERRAN, J. B., and C. DOW: Growth of Aujeszky's virus in rabbits and tissue cultures. Brit. vet. J. **118**, 386—389 (1962).

McFERRAN, J. B., and C. DOW: The excretion of Aujeszky's disease virus by experimentally infected pigs. Res. Vet. Sci. **5**, 405—410 (1964a).

McFERRAN, J. B., and C. DOW: Virus studies on experimental Aujeszky's disease in cattle. J. comp. Path. **74**, 173—179 (1964b).

McFERRAN, J. B., and C. DOW: The distribution of the virus of Aujeszky's disease (pseudorabies virus) in experimentally infected swine. Amer. J. vet. Res. **26**, 631—635 (1965).

MELNICK, J. L., and D. D. BANKER: Isolation of B virus (herpes group) from the central nervous system of a rhesus monkey. J. exp. Med. 100, 181–194 (1954).

MELNICK, J. L., and R. M. McCOMBS: Classification and nomenclature of animal viruses, 1966. Progr. med. Virol. 8, 400–409 (1966).

MESELSON, M., and F. W. STAHL: The replication of DNA in Escherichia coli. Proc. nat. Acad. Sci. (Wash.) 44, 671–682 (1958).

MESELSON, M., F. W. STAHL, and J. VINOGRAD: Equilibrium sedimentation of macromolecules in density gradients. Proc. nat. Acad. Sci. (Wash.) 43, 581–583 (1957).

MILLER, J. K., F. HESSER, and V. N. TOMPKINS: Herpes simplex encephalitis. Ann. intern. Med. 64, 92–103 (1966).

MITCHELL, J. E., and F. C. McCALL: Transplacental infection by herpes simplex virus. Amer. J. Dis. Child. 106, 207–209 (1963).

MORGAN, C., S. A. ELLISON, H. M. ROSE, and D. H. MOORE: Electron microscopic examination of inclusion bodies of herpes simplex virus. Proc. Soc. exp. Biol. (N.Y.) 82, 454–457 (1953).

MORGAN, C., S. A. ELLISON, H. M. ROSE, and D. H. MOORE: Structure and development of viruses as observed in the electron microscope. I. Herpes simplex virus. J. exp. Med. 100, 195–202 (1954).

MORGAN, C., E. P. JONES, M. HOLDEN, and H. M. ROSE: Intranuclear crystals of herpes simplex virus observed with the electron microscope. Virology 5, 568–571 (1958).

MORGAN, C., H. M. ROSE, M. HOLDEN, and E. P. JONES: Electron microscopic observations on the development of herpes simplex virus. J. exp. Med. 110, 643–656 (1959).

MORGAN, H. R., and M. FINLAND: Isolation of herpes virus from a case of atypical pneumonia and erythema multiforme exudativum with studies of four additional cases. Amer. J. med. Sci. 217, 92–95 (1949).

MUNK, K., and W. W. ACKERMANN: Some properties of herpes simplex virus. J. Immunol. 71, 425–430 (1953).

MUNK, K., und D. DONNER: Cytopathischer Effekt und Plaquemorphologie verschiedener Herpes-simplex-Virus-Stämme. Arch. ges. Virusforsch. 13, 529–540 (1963).

MUNK, K., und H. FISCHER: Fluoreszenzimmunologische Unterschiede bei Herpes-simplex-Virus-Stämmen. Arch. ges. Virusforsch. 15, 539–548 (1965).

MUNK, K., und G. SAUER: Autoradiographische Untersuchungen über das Verhalten der Desoxyribonucleinsäure in Herpesvirus-infizierten Zellen. Z. Naturforsch. 18b, 211–215 (1963).

MUNK, K., and G. SAUER: Relationship between cell DNA metabolism and nucleo-cytoplasmic alterations in herpes virus-infected cells. Virology 22, 153–154 (1964).

NACHKOV, D., L. CHRISTOPHOROV, C. GUÉNEV et V. STOYANOV: La réaction de fixation du complément dans la maladie d'Aujeszky chez les porcs. Off. Int. Epiz. 49, 383–388 (1958).

NAGLER, F. P. O.: A specific cutaneous reaction in persons infected with the virus of herpes simplex. J. Immunol. 48, 213–219 (1944).

NAHMIAS, A. J., S. KIBRICK, and P. BERNFIELD: Effect of synthetic and biological polyanions on herpes simplex virus. Proc. Soc. exp. Biol. (N.Y.) 115, 993–996 (1964).

NAHMIAS, A. J., S. KIBRICK, and R. C. ROSAN: Virus leucocyte interrelationships. I. Multiplication of a DNA virus — herpes simplex — in human leucocyte cultures. J. Immunol. 93, 69–74 (1964).

NANKERVIS, G. A., T. A. GRAY, and H. R. MORGAN: Host-virus relationships in Rous sarcoma tissues in vitro. II. Growth of extraneous viruses in Rous sarcoma and adult chick cells in vitro. J. nat. Cancer Inst. 22, 283–295 (1959).

NEWTON, A., P. P. DENDY, C. L. SMITH, and P. WILDY: A pool size problem associated with the use of tritiated thymidine. Nature (Lond.) 194. 886–887 (1962).

NEWTON, A., and M. G. P. STOKER: Changes in nucleic acid content of HeLa cells infected with herpes virus. Virology 5, 549—560 (1958).

NICOLAU, S.: Herpes, in "Les Ultravirus des Maladies Humaines" (LEVADITI et LÉPINE, eds). Vol. I, pp. 445—513, Paris: Libraire Maloine. 1948.

NII, S.: The difference in the cytopathic changes in FL cells infected with different strains of herpes simplex virus. Biken J. 4, 215—216 (1961).

NII, S., and J. KAMAHORA: Cytopathic changes induced by herpes simplex virus. Biken J. 4, 255—270 (1961).

NII, S., and J. KAMAHORA: Location of herpetic viral antigen in interphase cells. Biken J. 6, 145—154 (1963).

NOHARA, H., and A. S. KAPLAN: Induction of a new enzyme in rabbit kidney cells by pseudorabies virus. Biochem. biophys. Res. Commun. 12, 189—193 (1963).

NOJIMA, T.: A mutant of herpes simplex virus possessing an attenuated pathogenicity for baby mice obtained by egg passage of a newly-isolated strain. Jap. J. med. Sci. Biol. 13, 179—189 (1960).

NORCROSS, C., J. F. McCREA, and S. ANGERER: Purification of herpes simplex virus with fluorocarbon and potassium tartrate density gradients. Virology 21, 522—525 (1963).

NOVIKOFF, A. B.: Lysosomes in the physiology and pathology of cells contributions of staining methods. in "Lysosomes", Ciba Foundation Symposium (DE REUCH and CAMERON, eds.), pp. 36—73, Boston, Massachussets: Little, Brown and Co., 1963.

OLANDER, H. J., J. R. SAUNDERS, D. P. GUSTAFSON, and R. K. JONES: Pathologic findings in swine affected with a virulent strain of Aujeszky's virus. Path. Vet. 3, 64—82 (1966).

OSTERHOUT, S., and I. TAMM: Measurements of herpes simplex virus by the plaque technique in human amnion cells. J. Immunol. 83, 442—447 (1959).

PAINE, T. F., Jr.: Latent herpes simplex infection in man. Bact. Rev. 28, 472—479 (1964).

PATTERSON, A., A. D. FOX, G. DAVIES, C. MAGUIRE, P. J. HOME-SELLERS, P. WRIGHT, N. S. C. RICE, B. COBB, and B. R. JONES: Controlled studies of IDU in the treatment of herpetic keratitis. Trans. ophthal. Soc. U.K. 83, 583—591 (1963).

PAYROU, P., and C. H. DOHLMAN: IDU in corneal wound healing. Amer. J. Ophthal. 57, 999—1002 (1964).

PELMONT, J., et H. R. MORGAN: Facteurs nutritifs influençant la croissance du virus de l'herpès dans la souche de cellules L de Earle. Ann. Inst. Pasteur 96, 448—454 (1959).

PETTE, J.: Procédés modernes de diagnostic de la maladie d'Aujeszky. Bull. Off. Int. Epiz. 63, 1835—1851 (1965).

PFAU, C. J., and J. F. McCREA: Studies on the deoxyribonucleic acid of vaccinia virus. III. Characterization of DNA isolated by different methods and its relation to virus structure. Virology 21, 425—435 (1963).

PFEFFERKORN, E. R., B. W. BURGE, and H. M. COADY: Characteristics of the photoreactivation of pseudorabies virus. J. Bact. 92, 856—861 (1966).

PFEFFERKORN, E. R., C. RUTSTEIN, and B. W. BURGE: Photoreactivation of pseudorabies virus. Virology 27, 457—459 (1965).

PLATT, H.: The local and generalized forms of experimental herpes simplex infection in guinea pigs. Brit. J. exp. Path. 45, 300—308 (1964).

PLUMMER, G.: Serological comparison of the herpes viruses. Brit. J. exp. Path. 45, 135—141 (1964).

PLUMMER, G., and B. LEWIS: Thermoinactivation of herpes simplex virus and cytomegalovirus. J. Bact. 89, 671—674 (1965).

PLUMMER, G., and A. P. WATERSON: Equine herpes viruses. Virology 19, 412—416 (1963).

POLACK, F. M., and J. ROSE: The effect of 5-iodo-2'-deoxyuridine (IDU) in corneal healing. Arch. Ophthal. 71, 520—527 (1964).

POLLARD, E.: The action of ionizing radiation on viruses. Advanc. Virus Res. 2, 109—151 (1954).

POTTER, V. R.: Biochemical approach to the cancer problem. Fed. Proc. **17**, 691—
697 (1958).

POTTER, V. R.: In "Nucleic Acid Outlines", Vol. I, Minneapolis, Minnesota: Burgess.
1960.

POWELL, W. F.: Radiosensitivity as an index of herpes simplex virus development.
Virology **9**, 1—19 (1959).

PRUSOFF, W. H., Y. S. BAHKLE, and L. SEKELY: Cellular and antiviral effects of
halogenated deoxyribonucleosides. Ann. N. Y. Acad. Sci. **130**, 135—150 (1965).

PUGH, R. C. B., J. A. DUDGEON, and M. J. BODIAN: Kaposi's varicelliform eruption
(eczema herpeticum) with typical and atypical visceral necrosis. J. Path. Bact. **69**,
67—80 (1955).

RAPP, F.: Variants of herpes simplex virus: isolation, characterization, and factors
influencing plaque formation. J. Bact. **86**, 985—991 (1963).

RAPP, F., and T. C. HSU: Viruses and mammalian chromosomes. IV. Replication of
herpes simplex virus in diploid Chinese hamster cells. Virology **25**, 401—411
(1965).

RAWLS, W. E., P. J. DYCK, D. W. KLASS, H. D. GREER III, and E. C. HERRMANN, Jr.:
Encephalitis associated with herpes simplex virus. Ann. intern. Med. **64**, 104—
115 (1966).

RAY, J. D.: Pseudorabies (Aujeszky's disease) in suckling pigs in the United States.
Vet. Med. **38**, 178—179 (1943).

REISSIG, M., and A. S. KAPLAN: The induction of amitotic nuclear division by pseudorabies virus multiplying in single rabbit kidney cells. Virology **11**, 1—11 (1960).

REISSIG, M., and A. S. KAPLAN: The morphology of noninfective pseudorabies virus
produced by cells treated with 5-fluorouracil. Virology **16**, 1—8 (1962).

REISSIG, M., and J. L. MELNICK: The cellular changes produced in tissue cultures
by herpes B virus correlated with the concurrent multiplication of the virus. J.
exp. Med. **101**, 341—351 (1955).

REMLINGER, P., et J. BAILLY: Contribution à l'étude du virus herpétique (souche
marocaine). Ann. Inst. Pasteur **41**, 1314—1329 (1927).

REMLINGER, P., et J. BAILLY: Le siège du virus dans la maladie d'Aujeszky expérimentale. C. R. Soc. Biol. (Paris) **113**, 125—126 (1933).

ROGERS, A. M., L. L. CORIELL, H. BLANK, and T. F. McN. SCOTT: Acute herpetic
gingivostomatitis in the adult. New Engl. J. Med. **241**, 330—333 (1949).

ROIZMAN, B.: Virus infection of cells in mitosis. I. Observations on the recruitment of
cells in karyokinesis into giant cells induced by herpes simplex virus and bearing
on the site of virus antigen formation. Virology **13**, 387—401 (1961).

ROIZMAN, B.: The role of hormones in viral infections. II. Acceleration of viral adsorption and penetration into cells treated with thyroid hormone in vitro. Proc.
nat. Acad. Sci. (Wash.) **48**, 973—977 (1962).

ROIZMAN, B.: The programming of herpes virus multiplication in doubly-infected
and in puromycin-treated cells. Proc. nat. Acad. Sci. (Wash.) **49**, 165—171 (1963).

ROIZMAN, B.: Abortive infection of canine cells by herpes simplex virus. III. The
interference of conditional lethal mutants with an extended host range mutant.
Virology **27**, 113—117 (1965).

ROIZMAN, B., and L. AURELIAN: Abortive infection of canine cells by herpes simplex virus. I. Characterization of viral progeny from cooperative infection with
mutants differing in capacity to multiply in canine cells. J. molec. Biol. **11**, 528—
538 (1965).

ROIZMAN, B., G. S. BORMAN, and M.-K. ROUSTA: Macromolecular synthesis in cells
infected with herpes simplex virus. Nature (Lond.) **206**, 1374—1375 (1965).

ROIZMAN, B., and P. R. ROANE, Jr.: A physical difference between two strains of
herpes simplex virus apparent on sedimentation in cesium chloride. Virology **15**,
75—79 (1961).

ROIZMAN, B., and P. R. ROANE, Jr.: Demonstration of a surface difference between
virions of two strains of herpes simplex virus. Virology **19**, 198—204 (1963).

ROIZMAN, B., and P. R. ROANE, Jr.: The multiplication of herpes simplex virus. II. The relation between protein synthesis and the duplication of viral DNA in infected HEp-2 cells. Virology **22**, 262—269 (1964).

ROSS, R. W., and E. ORLANS: The redistribution of nucleic acid and the appearance of specific antigen in HeLa cells infected with herpes virus. J. Path. Bact. **76**, 393—402 (1958).

ROSS, C. A. C., W. C. RUSSELL, and P. WILDY: Herpes antigens from hamster kidney cell cultures in the diagnosis of primary and recurrent infections. Arch. ges. Virusforsch. **15**, 58—66 (1964).

RUBIN, H., M. BALUDA, and J. E. HOTCHIN: The maturation of Western equine encephalomyelitis virus and its release from chick embryo cells in suspension. J. exp. Med. **101**, 205—212 (1955).

RUCHMAN, I., and K. DODD: Recovery of herpes simplex from the blood of a patient with herpetic rhinitis. J. Lab. clin. Med. **35**, 434—439 (1950).

RUPERT, C. S.: Photoenzymatic repair of ultraviolet damage in DNA. I. Kinetics of reaction. J. gen. Physiol. **45**, 707—724 (1962a).

RUPERT, C. S.: Photoenzymatic repair of ultraviolet damage in DNA. II. Formation of an enzyme-substrate complex. J. gen. Physiol. **45**, 725—741 (1962b).

RUPERT, C. S., S. H. GOODGAL, and R. M. HERRIOTT: Photoreactivation *in vitro* of ultraviolet inactivated hemophilus influenzae transforming factor. J. gen. Physiol. **41**, 451—471 (1958).

RUPPE, J. P., Jr., E. F. WILSON, Jr., and W. WOLENS: Treatment of eczema herpeticum with gamma globulin. Arch. Derm. **76**, 572—574 (1957).

RUSSELL, W. C.: Herpes virus nucleic acid. Virology **16**, 355—357 (1962a).

RUSSELL, W. C.: A sensitive and precise plaque assay for herpes virus. Nature (Lond.) **195**, 1028—1029 (1962b).

RUSSELL, W. C., and L. V. CRAWFORD: Some characteristics of the deoxyribonucleic acid from herpes simplex virus. Virology **21**, 353—361 (1963).

RUSSELL, W. C., and L. V. CRAWFORD: Properties of the nucleic acids from some herpes group viruses. Virology **22**, 288—292 (1964).

RUSSELL, W. C., E. GOLD, H. M. KEIR, H. OMURA, D. H. WATSON, and P. WILDY: The growth of herpes simplex virus and its nucleic acid. Virology **22**, 103—110 (1964).

RUSSELL, W. C., D. H. WATSON, and P. WILDY: Preliminary chemical studies on herpes virus. Biochem. J. **87**, 26—27P (1963).

RUSTIGIAN, R., J. B. SMULOW, M. TYE, W. A. GIBSON, and E. SHINDELL: Studies on latent infection of skin and oral mucosa in individuals with recurrent herpes simplex. J. invest. Derm. **47**, 218—221.

SABIN, A.: The immunological relationships of pseudorabies (infectious bulbar paralysis, mad itch). Brit. J. exp. Path. **15**, 372—380 (1934).

SANGIORGI, G.: La filtrabilità del virus della pseudorabbia. Pathologica **6**, 201—204 (1914).

SAUNDERS, J. R., and D. P. GUSTAFSON: Serological and experimental studies of pseudorabies in swine. Proc. 68th Ann. Meeting U.S. Livestock Sanitary Ass., pp. 256—265 (1964).

SAUNDERS, J. R., D. P. GUSTAFSON, H. J. OLANDER, and R. K. JONES: An unusual outbreak of Aujeszky's disease in swine. 67th Ann. Proc. U.S. Livestock Sanitary Ass. pp. 331—346 (1963).

SCHERER, W. F.: The utilization of a pure strain of mammalian cells (Earle) for the cultivation of viruses *in vitro*. I. Multiplication of pseudorabies and herpes simplex viruses. Amer. J. Path. **29**, 113—137 (1953).

SCHERER, W. F., and J. T. SYVERTON: The viral range *in vitro* of a malignant human epithelial cell (strain HeLa, Gey). I. Multiplication of herpes simplex, pseudorabies, and vaccinia viruses. Amer. J. Path. **30**, 1057—1073 (1954).

SCHLESINGER, R. W.: Interference between animal viruses, *in* "The Viruses" (BURNET and STANLEY, eds.), vol. 3, pp. 157—194. New York—London: Academic Press. 1959.

Schmidt, J. R., and A. F. Rasmussen, Jr.: The influence of environmental temperature on the course of experimental herpes simplex infection. J. infect. Dis. **107**, 356—360 (1960a).

Schmidt, J. R., and A. F. Rasmussen, Jr.: Activation of latent herpes simplex encephalitis by chemical means. J. infect. Dis. **106**, 154—158 (1960b).

Schmidt, N. J., and E. H. Lennette: A colorimetric neutralization for herpes simplex virus, with observation on neutralizing and complement-fixing antibody levels in human sera. J. Immunol. **86**, 137—145 (1961).

Schmidt, N. J., E. H. Lennette, and C. W. Shon: A complement-fixing antigen for herpes simplex derived from chick-embryo tissue cultures. Amer. J. Hyg. **72**, 59—72 (1960).

Schmiedhoffer, J.: Pathologie der infektiösen Bulbär-Paralyse (Aujeszky'schen Krankheit). Z. Infekt.-Kr. Haustiere 8, 383—405 (1910).

Schneck, J. M.: The psychological component in a case of herpes simplex. Psychosom. Med. 9, 62—64 (1947).

Schneweis, K. E.: Über die Haltbarkeit von drei Herpes simplex Virus-Stämmen bei tiefen Temperaturen. Z. Hyg. Infekt.-Kr. 147, 319—326 (1961).

Schneweis, K. E.: Zum antigenen Aufbau des Herpes simplex Virus. Z. Immunforsch. **124**, 173—196 (1962a).

Schneweis, K. E.: Serologische Untersuchungen zur Typendifferenzierung des Herpesvirus hominis. Z. Immun.-Forsch. **124**, 24—28 (1962b).

Schneweis, K. E.: Die serologischen Beziehungen der Typen 1 und 2 von Herpesvirus hominis zu Herpesvirus simiae. Z. Immun.-Forsch. **124**, 337—341 (1962c).

Schofield, C. B. S.: The treatment of herpes progenitalis with 5-iodo-2'-deoxyuridine. Brit. J. Derm. **76**, 465—470 (1964).

Schur, V. A., and A. W. Holmes: Virus susceptibility of marmoset kidney cultures. Proc. Soc. exp. Biol. (N.Y.) **119**, 950—952 (1965).

Scott, L. V., F. G. Felton, and J. A. Barney: Hemagglutination with herpes simplex virus. J. Immunol. **78**, 211—213 (1957).

Scott, T. F. McN.: Epidemiology of herpetic infections. Amer. J. Ophthal. **43**, 134—146 (1957).

Scott, T. F. McN.: Arboviruses and herpes group viruses. Discussion. pp. 287—288. First International Conference on Vaccines Against Viral and Rickettsial Diseases of Man. Wld Hlth Org., Washington, D. C. (1967).

Scott, T. F. McN., H. Blank, L. L. Coriell, and H. Crouse: Pathology and pathogenesis of the cutaneous lesions of variola, vaccinia, herpes simplex, herpes zoster, and varicella. in "The Pathogenesis and Pathology of Viral Diseases" (Kidd, ed.), pp. 74—78. New York: Columbia University Press. 1950.

Scott, T. F. McN., C. F. Burgoon, L. L. Coriell, and H. Blank: The growth curve of the virus of herpes simplex in rabbit corneal cells grown in tissue culture with parallel observations on the development of the intranuclear inclusion body. J. Immunol. **71**, 385—396 (1953).

Scott, T. F. McN., L. Coriell, H. Blank, and C. F. Burgoon: Some comments on herpetic infection in children with special emphasis on unusual clinical manifestations. J. Pediat. **41**, 835—943 (1952).

Scott, T. F. McN., and D. L. McLeod: Cellular responses to infection with strains of herpes simplex virus. Ann. N.Y. Acad. Sci. **81**, 118—128 (1959).

Scott, T. F. McN., D. L. McLeod, and T. Tokumaru: A biologic comparison of two strains of Herpesvirus hominis. J. Immunol. **86**, 1—12 (1961).

Scott, T. F. McN., A. J. Steigman, and J. H. Convey: Acute infectious gingivostomatitis. Etiology, epidemiology and clinical picture of a common disorder caused by the virus of herpes simplex. J. Amer. med. Ass. **117**, 999—1005 (1951).

Scott, T. F. McN., and T. Tokumaru: The herpesvirus group. in "Viral and Rickettsial Infections of Man" (Horsfall and Tamm, eds.) 4th edition, pp. 892—914. Philadelphia: J. B. Lippincott Company. 1965.

Seidenberg, S.: Zur Ätiologie der Pustulosis vacciniformis acuta. Schweiz. Z. allg. Path. **4**, 398—401 (1941).

SERY, T. W., and F. P. FURGIUELE: The inactivation of herpes simplex virus by chemical agents. Amer. J. Ophthal. **51**, 42—57 (1961).

SETLOW, R. B., and J. K. SETLOW: Evidence that ultraviolet-induced thymine dimers in DNA cause biological damage. Proc. nat. Acad. Sci. (Wash.) **48**, 1250—1257 (1962).

SHAHAN, M. S., R. L. KNUDSON, H. R. SEIBOLD, and C. N. DALE: Aujeszky's disease (pseudorabies). A review, with notes on two strains of the virus. N. Amer. Vet. **28**, 440—449; 511—521 (1947).

SHARON, N.: Stimulation of herpes simplex virus propagation in WISH cells by arginine. IXth International Congress for Microbiology, Abstracts of Papers, p. 508 (1966).

SHOPE, R. E.: An experimental study of mad itch with special reference to its relationship to pseudorabies. J. exp. Med. **45**, 233—248 (1931).

SHOPE, R. E.: Identity of the viruses causing "mad itch" and pseudorabies. Proc. Soc. exp. Biol. (N.Y.) **30**, 308—309 (1932).

SHOPE, R. E.: Experiments on the epidemiology of pseudorabies. I. Mode of transmission of the disease in swine and their possible role in its spread to cattle. J. exp. Med. **62**, 85—99 (1935a).

SHOPE, R. E.: Experiments on the epidemiology of pseudorabies. II. Prevalence of the disease among Middle Western swine and the possible role of rats in herd to herd infections. J. exp. Med. **62**, 101—117 (1935b).

SHOPE, R. E.: Pseudorabies (Aujeszky's disease, mad itch, infectious bulbar paralysis). *in* "Diseases in Swine" (DUNNE, ed.), 2nd edition, The Iowa State University Press. 1964.

SHUBLADZE, A. K., T. M. MAEVSKAIA, V. A. ANAN'EV, and V. N. VOLKOVA: On some features of different strains of herpes viruses. I. Antigenic properties. Vop. Virus. **5**, 735—740 (1960).

SIGEL, M. M.: Influence of age on susceptibility to virus infections with particular reference to laboratory animals. Ann. Rev. Microbiol. **6**, 257—280 (1952).

SINGH, K. V.: A plaque assay of pseudorabies virus in monolayers of porcine kidney cells. Cornell Vet. **52**, 237—246 (1962).

SINSHEIMER, R. L.: A single-stranded deoxyribonucleic acid from bacteriophage $\bigcirc$X 174. J. molec. Biol. **1**, 43—53 (1959).

ŠKODA, R.: A modified pseudorabies virus suitable for immunization of cattle. Acta virol. **6**, 189 (1962).

ŠKODA, R., I. BRAUNER, E. SÁDECKÝ, and V. MAYER: Immunization against Aujeszky's disease with live vaccine. I. Attenuation of virus and some properties of attenuated strains. Acta virol. **8**, 1—9 (1964).

ŠKODA, R., I. BRAUNER, E. SÁDECKÝ, and J. SOMOGYIOVÁ: Immunization against Aujeszky's disease with live virus. II. Immunization of pigs under laboratory conditions. Acta virol. **8**, 123—134 (1964).

ŠKODA, R., I. BRAUNER, E. SÁDECKÝ, J. SOMOGYIOVÁ, and O. JAMRICHOVÁ: Immunization against Aujeszky's disease with a live vaccine. III. Immunization of pigs with the vaccine BUK in field conditions. Vet. Med. **11**, 85—95 (1966).

ŠKODA, R., und Z. GRUNERT: Epizootologie der Aujeszky'schen Krankheit in der ČSSR. I. Mitteilung: Geschichte des Vorkommens und geographische Verbreitung. Arch. exp. Vet.-Med. **19**, 577—585 (1965).

ŠKODA, R., and O. JAMRICHOVÁ: Small plaque variants of pseudorabies virus in chick embryo cell cultures. Acta virol. **9**, 94 (1965).

ŠKODA, R., E. SÁDECKÝ und J. MOLNÁR: Über die bei Mutterschweinen nach natürlicher Infektion serologisch nachweisbare Immunität gegen die Aujeszky'sche Krankheit. Arch. exp. Vet.-Med. **17**, 1363—1370 (1963).

ŠKODA, R., und A. ŽUFFA: Die Diagnostik der Aujeszky'schen Krankheit in Gewebekulturen. Arch. exp. Vet.-Med. **16**, 491—500 (1962).

SLAVIN, H. B., and G. P. BERRY: Studies on herpetic infection in mice. II. Pathway of invasion of the central nervous system after intranasal instillation of virus in suckling mice. J. exp. Med. **68**, 315—320 (1943).

SLAVIN, H. B., and E. GAVETT: Primary herpetic vulvovaginitis. Proc. Soc. exp. Biol.
    (N.Y.) 63, 343—345 (1946a).
SLAVIN, H. B., and E. GAVETT: Antigenic dissimilarity between strains of herpes
    simplex virus. Proc. Soc. exp. Biol. (N.Y.) 63, 345—347 (1964b).
SMITH, K. O.: Some biologic aspects of herpesvirus — cell interactions in the presence
    of 5-iodo-2'-deoxyuridine (IDU). Demonstration of a cytotoxic effect by herpes-
    viruses. J. Immunol. 91, 582—590 (1963).
SMITH, K. O.: Relationship between the envelope and the infectivity of herpes sim-
    plex virus. Proc. Soc. exp. Biol. (N.Y.) 115, 814—816 (1964).
SMITH, K. O., and C. B. DUKES: Effects of 5-iodo-2'-deoxyuridine (IDU) on herpes
    virus synthesis and survival in infected cells. J. Immunol. 92, 550—554 (1964).
SMITH, K. O., and J. L. MELNICK: Recognition and quantitation of herpesvirus parti-
    cles in human vesicular lesions. Science 137, 543—544 (1962).
SOMERS, C. E., and T. C. HSU: Chromosome damage induced by hydroxylamine
    in mammalian cells. Proc. nat. Acad. Sci. (Wash.) 48, 937—953 (1962).
SOMOGYIOVÁ, J.: Persistent pseudorabies virus infection of primary calf kidney cell
    cultures. Acta virol. 9, 557 (1965).
SOSA-MARTINEZ, J., L. GUTIERREZ-VILLEGAS, and R. M. SOSA: Propagation of
    herpes simplex virus in tissue cultures of rabbit kidney cells. J. Bact. 70, 391—
    399 (1955).
SOSA-MARTINEZ, J., e E. H. LENNETTE: Sobre un antigeno soluble del herpes simple.
    Ciencia (Méx.) 19, 249—258 (1959).
SPEAR, P. G., and B. ROIZMAN: Buoyant density of herpes simplex virus in solutions
    of caesium chloride. Nature (Lond.) 214, 713—714 (1967).
SPECK, R. S., E. JAWETZ, and V. R. COLEMAN: Studies on herpes simplex virus. I.
    The stability and preservation of egg-adapted herpes simplex virus. J. Bact. 61,
    253—258 (1951).
SPRING, S. B., and B. ROIZMAN: Herpes simplex virus products in productive and
    abortive infection. I. Stabilization with formaldehyde and preliminary analyses
    by isopycnic centrifugation in CsCl. J. Virol. 1, 294—301 (1967).
STEVENS, J. G., and N. B. GROMAN: Properties of infectious bovine rhinotracheitis
    virus in a quantitated virus-cell culture system. Amer. J. vet. Res. 24, 1158—1163
    (1963).
STICH, H. F., T. C. HSU, and F. RAPP: Viruses and mammalian chromosomes. I.
    Localization of chromosome aberrations after infection with herpes simplex virus.
    Virology 22, 439—445 (1964).
STOKER, M. G. P.: Growth studies with herpes virus. Ninth Symposium Soc. gen.
    Microbiol. pp. 142—170 (1959).
STOKER, M. G. P., and A. NEWTON: The effect of herpes virus on HeLa cells dividing
    parasynchronously. Virology 7, 438—448 (1959).
STOKER, M. G. P., and R. W. ROSS: Quantitative studies on the growth of herpes
    virus in HeLa cells. J. gen. Microbiol. 19, 250—267 (1958).
STOKER, M. G. P., K. M. SMITH, and R. W. ROSS: Electron microscopic studies of
    HeLa cells infected with herpes virus. J. gen. Microbiol. 19, 244—249 (1958).
STOLLAR, D., and L. GROSSMAN: The reaction of formaldehyde with denatured
    DNA: spectrophotometric, immunologic, and enzymic studies. J. molec. Biol. 4,
    31—38 (1962).
STULBERG, C. S., and R. SCHAPIRA: Virus growth in tissue culture fibroblasts. I.
    Influenza A and herpes simplex viruses. J. Immunol. 70, 51—59 (1953).
SUBAK-SHARPE, H., R. R. BÜRK, L. V. CRAWFORD, J. M. MORRISON, J. HAY, and
    H. M. KEIR: An approach to evolutionary relationships of mammalian DNA
    viruses through analysis of the pattern of nearest neighbor base sequences. Cold
    Spr. Harb. Symp. quant. Biol. 31, 737—748 (1966a).
SUBAK-SHARPE, H., and J. HAY: An animal virus with DNA of high guanine +
    cytosine content which codes for s-RNA. J. molec. Biol. 12, 924—928 (1965).
SUBAK-SHARPE, H., W. M. SHEPHERD, and J. HAY: Studies on sRNA coded by
    herpes virus. Cold Spr. Harb. Symp. quant. Biol. 31, 583—594 (1966b).

SUEOKA, N., J. MARMUR, and P. DOTY: Heterogeneity in deoxyribonucleic acids. II. Dependence of the density of deoxyribonucleic acids on guanine + cytosine content. Nature (Lond.) **183**, 1429—1431 (1959).

SYDISKIS, R. J., and B. ROIZMAN: Polysomes and protein synthesis in cells infected with a DNA virus. Science **153**, 76—78 (1966).

SYVERTON, J. T., and G. P. BERRY: Multiple virus infection of single host cells. J. exp. Med. **86**, 145—152 (1947).

SZÁNTÓ, J.: Stable cell strains from rabbit and lung tissue suitable for the propagation of herpes simplex virus. Acta virol. **4**, 380—382 (1960).

SZÁNTÓ, J.: Course of persistent infection of HeLa and Detroit 6 cells with herpes simplex virus. Acta virol. **7**, 385—392 (1963).

TAKEMOTO, K. K., and P. FABISCH: Inhibition of herpes virus by natural and synthetic polysaccharides. Proc. Soc. exp. Biol. (N.Y.) **116**, 140—144 (1964).

TALAL, N., G. M. TOMKINS, J. F. MUSHINSKI, and K. L. YIELDING: Immunochemical evidence for multiple molecular forms of crystalline glutamine dehydrogenase. J. molec. Biol. **8**, 46—53 (1964).

TANIGUCHI, S., and K. YOSHINO: Studies on the neutralization of herpes simplex virus. II. Analysis of complement as the antibody potentiating factor. Virology **26**, 54—60 (1965).

TANKERSLEY, R. W., Jr.: Amino acid requirements of herpes simplex virus in human cells. J. Bact. **87**, 609—613 (1964).

TANZER, J., M. THOMAS, Y. STOITCHKOV, M. BOIRON et J. BERNARD: Altérations chromosomiques observées dans les cellules de rein de singe infectées *in vitro* par le virus de l'herpès. Ann. Inst. Pasteur **107**, 366—372 (1964).

TATENO, I., T. YOKOYAMA, S. SUZUKI, A. SUGIURA, and I. FUKAYA: Age distribution of neutralizing antibody to herpes simplex virus. Jap. J. exp. Med. **28**, 375—380 (1958).

TAVERNE, J., and P. WILDY: Purification of herpes simplex virus by chromatography of calcium phosphate. Nature (Lond.) **184**, 1655—1656 (1959).

TERPSTRA, J. I.: Ze ziekte van Aujeszky bij varkens. T. Diergeneesk. **83**, 431—436 (1958).

THOMPSON, R. L., and M. S. COATES: The effect of temperature upon the growth and survival of myxoma, herpes, and vaccinia virus in tissue culture. J. infect. Dis. **71**, 83—85 (1942).

THYGESON, P.: Ocular viral diseases. Med. Clin. N. Amer. **43**, 1419—1440 (1959).

THYGESON, P., M. J. HOGAN, and S. J. KIMURA: Cortisone and hydrocortisone in ocular infections. Trans. Amer. Acad. Ophthal. Otolaryngol. **57**, 64—85 (1953).

TOKUMARU, T.: Pseudorabies virus in tissue culture: differentiation of two distinct strains of virus by cytopathogenic pattern induced. Proc. Soc. exp. Biol. (N.Y.) **96**, 55—60 (1957).

TOKUMARU, T., and T. F. McN. SCOTT: personal communication (1964).

TOKUMARU, T., and T. F. McN. SCOTT: The herpesvirus group: Herpesvirus hominis, Herpesvirus simiae, Herpesvirus suis. *In* "Diagnostic Procedures for Viral and Rickettsial Diseases" (LENNETTE and SCHMIDT, eds.). 3rd edition, pp. 381—433. New York: American Public Health Association. 1964.

TONEVA, V.: La maladie d'Aujeszky. Monograph, Sofia (1958).

TONEVA, V.: Obtention d'une souche non-virulente du virus de la maladie d'Aujeszky au moyen de passages et de l'adaptation des pigeons. C. R. Acad. bulgare Sci. **14**, 187—190 (1961).

TONEVA, V.: Purification et concentration du virus de la maladie d'Aujeszky par ultracentrifugation et chromatographie sur colonnes. Microscopie électronique du même virus. Clin. vet. (Milano) **88**, 289—315 (1965).

TOURNIER, P., and A. LWOFF: Systematics and nomenclature of viruses. The PCNV proposals. IXth International Congress for Microbiology, Symposia, pp. 417—422 (1966).

TRAINER, D. O., and L. KARSTAD: Experimental pseudorabies in some wild North American mammals. Zoonoses Res. **2**, 135—150 (1963).

TYTELL, A. A., and R. E. NEUMAN: A medium free of agar, serum and peptone for plaque assay of herpes simplex virus. Proc. Soc. exp. Biol. (N.Y.) 113, 343—346 (1963).

UNDERWOOD, G. E.: Activity of 1-β-D-arabinofuranosylcytosine hydrochloride against herpes simplex keratitis. Proc. Soc. exp. Biol. (N.Y.) 111, 660—664 (1962).

UNDERWOOD, G. E., G. A. ELLIOTT, and D. A. BUTHALA: Herpes keratitis in rabbits: pathogenesis and effect of antiviral nucleosides. Ann. N.Y. Acad. Sci. 130, 151—167 (1965).

UNDERWOOD, G. E., C. A. WISNER, and S. D. WEED: Cytosine arabinoside (CA) and other nucleosides in herpes virus infections. Arch. Ophthal. 72, 505—512 (1964).

URBAIN, A., et W. SCHAEFFER: Contribution a l'étude expérimentale d'un virus herpétique (souche Marocaine). Ann. Inst. Pasteur 43, 369—385 (1929).

VAHERI, A., and K. CANTELL: The effect of heparin on herpes simplex virus. Virology 21, 661—662 (1963).

VAN DER NOORDAA, J., J. F. ENDERS, and G. TH. DIAMANDOPOULOS: Increased resistance to herpes simplex virus of hamster and human cells transformed by SV40. Proc. Soc. exp. Biol. (N.Y.) 122, 915—920 (1966).

VAN ROOYEN, C. E., and A. J. RHODES: Virus Diseases of Man. New York: Thomas Nelson and Sons. 1948.

VIDAL, J. B.: Inoculabilité des pustules d'ecthyma. Ann. Derm. Syph. (Paris) 4, 350—358 (1873).

VON KERÉKJÁRTÓ, B., und B. RHODE: Über die Vermehrung des Aujeszky-Virus auf Affennieren-Epithelkulturen. Z. Naturforsch. 12b, 292—298 (1957).

WALLIS, C., and J. L. MELNICK: Irreversible photosensitization of viruses. Virology 23, 520—527 (1964).

WATERSON, A. P. C.: Plaque formation by herpes virus in chick embryo tissue. Arch. ges. Virusforsch. 8, 592—599 (1958).

WATKINS, J. F.: The early stages of infection of HeLa cells with herpes simplex virus. J. gen. Microbiol. 22, 57—71 (1960).

WATSON, D. H., W. C. RUSSELL, and P. WILDY: Electron microscopic particle counts on herpes virus using phosphotungstate negative staining technique. Virology 19, 250—260 (1963).

WATSON, D. H., and P. WILDY: Some serological properties of herpes virus particles studied with the electron microscope. Virology 21, 100—111 (1963).

WATSON, D. H., P. WILDY, B. A. M. HARVEY, and W. I. H. SHEDDEN: Serological relationships among viruses of the herpes group. J. gen. Virol. 1, 139—141 (1967).

WATSON, D. H., P. WILDY, and W. C. RUSSELL: Quantitative electron microscope studies on the growth of herpes virus using the techniques of negative staining and ultramicrotomy. Virology 24, 523—538 (1964).

WEISSMAN, S. M., R. M. S. SMELLIE, and J. PAUL: Studies on the biosynthesis of deoxyribonucleic acid by extracts of mammalian cells. IV. The phosphorylation of thymidine. Biochim. biophys. Acta (Amst.) 45, 101—110 (1960).

WENNER, H. A.: Complications of infantile eczema caused by the virus of herpes simplex. (a) Description of the clinical characteristics of an unusual eruption and (b) identification of an associated filterable virus. Amer. J. Dis. Child. 67, 247—264 (1944).

WEYER, E. R.: Herpes antiviral substances: Distribution in various age groups and apparent absence in individuals susceptible to poliomyelitis. Proc. Soc. exp. Biol. (N.Y.) 30, 309—313 (1932).

WHEELER, C. E.: The effect of temperature upon the production of herpes simplex virus in tissue culture. J. Immunol. 81, 98—106 (1958).

WHEELER, C. E.: Further studies on the effect of neutralizing antibody upon the course of herpes simplex infections in tissue culture. J. Immunol. 84, 394—40 (1960).

WHEELER, C. E.: Biologic comparison of a syncytial and a small giant cell-forming strain of herpes simplex. J. Immunol. 93, 749—756 (1964).

WHEELER, C. E., and W. D. HUFFINES: Primary disseminated herpes simplex of the newborn. J. Amer. med. Ass. 191, 455—460 (1965).

WHITE, D. O., and A. W. HARRIS: Actions of metal chelates of substituted 1, 10-phenanthrolines on viruses and cells. 1. Inactivation of viruses. Aust. J. exp. Biol. med. Sci. **41**, 517—526 (1963).

WHITEHOUSE, F., Jr., P. K. WILLIAMS, and H. F. FALLS: The effect of betaproprio-lactone on herpes simplex virus in vitro and in vivo. Univ. Mich. med. Bull. **27**—**28**, 388—397 (1961/62).

WIBERG, J. S., M. L. DIRKSEN, R. H. EPSTEIN, S. E. LURIA, and J. M. BUCHANAN: Early enzyme synthesis and its control in E. coli infected with some amber mutants of bacteriophage T4. Proc. nat. Acad. Sci. (Wash.) **48**, 293—302 (1962).

WILDY, P.: Path of herpes virus infection from the periphery to the central nervous system in mice. Quoted by F. M. BURNET *in* "Principles of Animal Virology", 1st edition, pp. 226—227, New York: Academic Press. Inc. 1955.

WILDY, P.: General principles of virus taxonomy. IXth International Congress for Microbiology, Symposia, pp. 433—439 (1966).

WILDY, P.: The progression of herpes simplex virus to the central nervous system of the mouse. J. Hyg. (Lond.) **65**, 173—192 (1967).

WILDY, P., and H. F. HOLDEN: The complement-fixing antigen of herpes simplex virus. Aust. J. exp. Biol. Med. Sci. **32**, 621—632 (1954).

WILDY, P., and R. W. HORNE: The structure of herpes simplex virus and its relation to other viruses. Proc. Eur. Reg. Conf. on Electron Microscopy, Delft **2**, 955—963 (1960).

WILDY, P., W. C. RUSSELL, and R. W. HORNE: The morphology of herpes virus. Virology **12**, 204—222 (1960).

WILDY, P., M. G. P. STOKER, and R. W. ROSS: Release of herpes virus from solitary HeLa cells. J. gen. Microbiol. **20**, 105—112 (1959).

WOLMAN, M., and A. J. BEHAR: Cytochemical evidence for the nature of herpes simplex inclusion bodies. J. infect. Dis. **91**, 63—68 (1952).

WOMACK, C. R., and B. P. HUNT: Serologic differences in strains of herpes simplex virus. Science **120**, 227—228 (1954).

WOMACK, C. R., and C. C. RANDALL: Erythema exudativum multiforme. Amer. J. Med. **15**, 633—644 (1953).

WRIGHT, B. E.: On enzyme-substrate relationships during biochemical differentiation. Proc. nat. Acad. Sci. (Wash.) **46**, 798—803 (1960).

YOSHINO, K., and S. TANIGUCHI: The appearance of complement-requiring neutralizing antibodies by immunization and infection with herpes simplex virus. Virology **22**, 193—201 (1964).

YOSHINO, K., and S. TANIGUCHI: Studies on the neutralization of herpes simplex virus. I. Appearance of neutralizing antibodies having different grades of complement requirement. Virology **26**, 44—53 (1965).

YOSHINO, K., and S. TANIGUCHI: Evaluation of the demonstration of complement-requiring neutralizing antibody as a means for early diagnosis of herpes virus infections. J. Immunol. **96**, 196—203 (1966).

YOSHINO, K., H. TANIGUCHI, and S. TANIGUCHI: Demonstration of the eclipse phase of herpes simplex virus by a new de-embryonation technique. Virology **10**, 97—111 (1960).

YOSHINO, K., S. TANIGUCHI, R. FURUSE, T. NOJIMA, R. FUJII, M. MINAMITANI, R. TADA, and H. KUBOTA: A serological survey for antibodies against herpes simplex virus with special reference to comparatively heat-labile complement-fixing antibodies. Jap. J. med. Sci. Biol. **15**, 235—247 (1962).

YOUNGNER, J. S.: Virus adsorption and plaque formation in monolayer cultures of trypsin-dispersed monkey kidney. J. Immunol. **76**, 288—292 (1956).

ZUELZER, W. W., and C. S. STULBERG: Herpes simplex virus as the cause of fulminating visceral disease and hepatitis in infancy. Amer. J. Dis. Child. **83**, 421—437 (1952).

ŽUFFA, A.: Immunisierung gegen die Aujeszky'sche Krankheit. I. Gewinnung des modifizierten Virus der Aujeszky'schen Krankheit. Arch. exp. Vet.-Med. **17**, 1325—1344 (1963).

ŽUFFA, A.: Immunisierung gegen die Aujeszky'sche Krankheit. Zbl. Bakt. I. Abt. Orig. **192**, 280—287 (1964).

VIROLOGY MONOGRAPHS

Prospekt steht zur Verfügung

DIE VIRUSFORSCHUNG IN EINZELDARSTELLUNGEN

Bisher erschienen:

Volume 1: ECHO Viruses

By Dr. H. A. WENNER and Dr. A. M. BEHBEHANI, Section for Virus Research, Department of Pediatrics, University of Kansas School of Medicine, Kansas City, Kansas, U.S.A.

Reoviruses

By Dr. L. ROSEN, Pacific Research Section, Laboratory of Infectious Diseases, National Institute of Allergy and Infectious Diseases, National Institutes of Health, U. S. Public Health Service, Honolulu, Hawaii, U.S.A.

With 4 figures. IV, 107 pages. 1968.
Cloth S 189.—, DM 30.—, US $ 7.50

Volume 2: The Simian Viruses

By Dr. R. N. HULL, The Lilly Research Laboratories, Indianapolis, Indiana, U.S.A.

Rhinoviruses

By Dr. D. A. J. TYRRELL, Clinical Research Centre, Common Cold Research Unit, Salisbury, Wiltshire, England.

With 19 figures. IV, 124 pages. 1968.
Cloth S 214.—, DM 34.—, US $ 8.50

Volume 3: Cytomegaloviruses

By Prof. Dr. J. B. HANSHAW, University of Rochester School of Medicine and Dentistry, Rochester, N.Y., U.S.A.

Rinderpest Virus

By Dr. W. PLOWRIGHT, East African Veterinary Research Organisation, Muguga, Kenya, E. Africa.

Lumpy Skin Disease Virus

By Dr. K. E. WEISS, Department of Agriculture, Division of Veterinary Service, Onderstepoort, Republic of South Africa.

With 26 figures. IV, 131 pages. 1968.
Cloth S 214.—, DM 34.—, US $ 8.50

Volume 4: The Influenza Viruses

By Dr. L. HOYLE, Public Health Laboratory, Northampton, England.

With 58 figures. IV, 375 pages. 1968.
Cloth S 680.—, DM 108.—, US $ 27.00

Weitere Bände in Vorbereitung

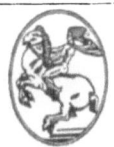 **SPRINGER-VERLAG**
WIEN · NEW YORK